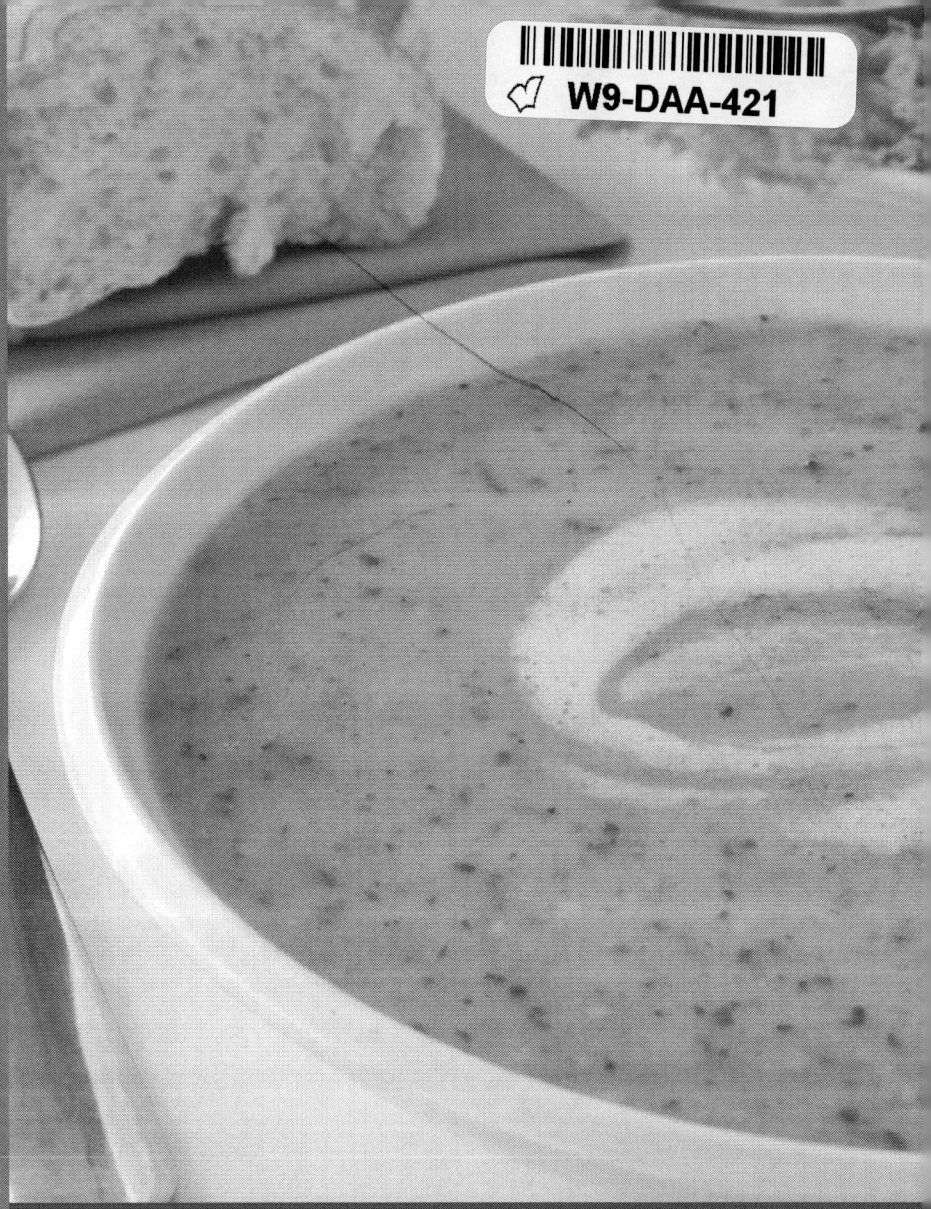

W9-DAA-421

The Dr. Gourmet Diet™ for Coumadin® Users

AN
CC 8117
$19.95
8/15

Dr. Gourmet

Timothy S. Harlan, M.D.

The Dr. Gourmet Diet for Coumadin Users

Copyright 2012 by Timothy S. Harlan, M.D.
All rights reserved. No part of this book shall be reproduced, stored in a retrieval system, or transmitted by any means - electronic, mechanical, photocopying, recording or otherwise - without written permission from the publisher. No Patent or medical liability is assumed with respect to the information contained herein. Although every precaution has been taken in the preparation of this book, the publisher and author assume no responsibility for errors or omissions. Nor is any liability assumed for damages resulting from the use of information contained herein.

Trademarks
All terms mentioned in this book that are known to be trademarks or service marks have been appropriately capitalized. Timothy S. Harlan, M.D. cannot attest to the accuracy of this information. Use of a term in this book should not be regarded as affecting the validity of any trademark or service mark.

The Dr. Gourmet name and Logo are trademarks of Timothy S. Harlan, M.D.. They are registered with the United States Patent and Trademark Office. All rights are reserved.

Terms of Use
The Content of this book and the Dr. Gourmet website, including recipes, nutrition and health information, text, graphics, images, calculators, columns and other material contained on the Dr. Gourmet website or in this book, is solely for informational purposes. Any communication with any staff member of the Dr. Gourmet website does not constitute a physician or health care provider / patient relationship.

Information on the Dr. Gourmet website or in this book should not be used in place of a visit or call to your doctor. You should not make changes in your medical therapy or any advice given to you by your physician without consulting them first.

The Content presented on the Dr. Gourmet website and in this book is not intended to be a substitute for professional medical advice. No effort is made at diagnosis or treatment of any condition. Only your doctor can help you with diagnosis and treatment of medical problems. Always discuss your concerns with your physician, asking any questions you may have regarding your medical condition. Do not disregard any advice given to you by any medical professional because of any information that you have read on the Dr. Gourmet website or in this book.

Table of Contents

Introduction **1**
How it Works 1
Prescribing Coumadin® (warfarin) 2
Interactions 2
Adjusting the Dose 3
Common Side Effects 3
Rash 3
Bleeding 3
Warfarin Necrosis 4
Purple Toe Syndrome 4
Osteoporosis 4
Contraindications 4
Other Interactions 4
Supplements 5
Vitamin K Dosage 5
Pictures of Coumadin® (warfarin) tablets 6
How to Use This Diet 6
Female 7
Male 7
More About the Recipes 8
The Rules 8
A word or two about what to drink 9
Breakfast Guidelines 10
Lunch Guidelines 12
Weekly Meal Plans - Coumadin® (warfarin) 13
Week One Menu and Grocery List 14
Week Two Menu and Grocery List 16
Week Three Menu and Grocery List 18
Week Four Menu and Grocery List 20
Week Five Menu and Grocery List 22
Week Six Menu and Grocery List 24
Recipes **27**
Breakfast Recipes 27
Apple Pancake 28
Blueberry Muffins 29

Scrambled Eggs 30
Blueberry Pancakes 31
Jean's French Toast 32
Zucchini and Chévre Frittata 33
Blueberry Blue Cornmeal Pancakes 34
Four Grain Pancakes 35
Tortilla 36
Orange French Toast 37
Orange Blueberry Scones 38
Pumpkin Nut Muffins 39
Omelet 40
Apple Cinnamon Bread 41
Salads 42
Curried Chicken Salad 42
Lentil and Black Bean Salad 43
Thai Cucumber Salad 44
Mediterranean Chicken Salad 45
Jicama Salad 46
Spaghetti Squash Salad 47
Roasted Eggplant Salad 48
Black Eyed Pea Salad 49
Main Course 50
Pizza with Tomato, Basil and Roasted Garlic 50
Whole Wheat Pizza Dough 51
Roasted Garlic 52
Butternut Squash Risotto 53
Seared Tuna Steak with Sake-Wasabi Sauce 54
Linguine with Shrimp in Vodka Tomato Cream Sauce 55
Fettuccine with Dill Pesto and Shrimp 56
Meatloaf 57
Roasted Salmon with Red Thai Curry 58
Indian Shrimp Curry 59
Mushroom Risotto 60
Roasted Salmon and Corn Relish 61
Corn Quesadillas 62
Jerk Shrimp 63
Jerk Rub 64

Chicken with Tarragon Mustard Cream 65
Halibut with Seven Spices 66
Mojo Pork Tenderloin 67
Tomato Saffron Risotto with Salmon 68
Oven Fried Chicken 69
Chili Rellenos 70
Creamy Mac and Cheese 71
Thai Coconut Shrimp 72
Salmon with Parmesan Crust 73
Fettuccine Alfredo 74
London Broil with Mushrooms Sautéed in Cognac 75
Philly Cheese Steak 76
Sea Bass with White Beans and Tomato Vinaigrette 77
Pepperoni Pizza 78
Pizza with Dill Pesto and Potato 79
Baked Penne 80
Barbecue Chicken 81
Ginger Cilantro Flank Steak 82
Pizza with Thai Peanut Sauce & Scallops 83
Grilled Sage Lamb Kabob 84
Gnocchi 85
Tomato Sauce 86
Mustard Seared Whitefish 87
Pan-Seared Pork Chops with Savory Peach Marmalade 88
Turkey Burgers 89
Extras 90
Cocktail Sauce 90
Thai Peanut Sauce 91
Roasted Garlic 92
Candied Carrots 93
Coconut Rice 94
Jasmine Rice 95
Herbed Zucchini 96
Green Beans with Walnut Vinaigrette 97
Roasted Garlic Mashed Potatoes 98
Green Beans with Red Onions 99
French Fries 100

Roasted Beets 101
Roasted Acorn Squash 102
Brown Rice 103
Plain Mashed Potatoes 104
Roasted Corn on the Cob 105
Parmesan Squash 106
Melon Salsa 107
Couscous 108
Rice and Lentil Pilaf 109
Dirty Rice 110
Mashed Yams 111
Zucchini with Sun Dried Tomatoes 112
Thick Cut Yam Fries 113

Soups 114

Beef Stew 114
Minestrone 115
Split Pea Soup 116
Creamy Chicken and Potato Soup 117
Lentil Soup 118

Ask Dr. Gourmet 119

Does salt increase INR levels? 120
Can I cook with parsley while on Coumadin? 120
Should I avoid lettuce while on Coumadin? 120
Can you wean down your dose of Coumadin? 121
Does Coumadin cause fatigue? 121
Does Coumadin® (warfarin) affect your metabolism and cause weight gain? 122
Should you avoid cranberry juice on Coumadin® (warfarin)? 122
Does alcohol interact with Coumadin? 123
Should I avoid caffeinated coffee on Coumadin® (warfarin)? 123
How much Vitamin K is in Fresca®, Sprite®, or other sodas? 123
If I'm on Coumadin, can I use Green Tea for weight loss? 124
Are there any documented problems with people drinking the supplement "Mona Vie" while on Coumadin? 125

Vitamin K Content of Foods 126

Short list 126

High (over 40 mcg Vitamin K per serving) 126
Medium (between 20 and 40 mcg Vitamin K per serving) 127
Comprehensive list 128

Introduction

Coumadin® (warfarin) is a prescription medication used for anticoagulation. It is often referred to as "a blood thinner," but that is not really an accurate description. It works by inhibiting enzymes that lead to blood clotting. It is the only well researched, effective oral medication for this purpose. (Other brand names for warfarin are Jantoven, Marevan, and Waran.)

Its primary use is to treat or prevent blood clots. When the blood clots in a vein or artery, physicians refer to it as a thrombus. When the thrombus breaks free and travels to other parts of the body it is known as an embolus. A common problem known as deep vein thrombosis (DVT) occurs when such clots form in the large veins in the legs or arms. These will commonly form and then break free and travel to the lungs, blocking blood flow, which is known as a pulmonary embolus (PE).

Other uses include:

- ✔ Pulmonary embolism
- ✔ Artificial heart valves
- ✔ Atrial fibrillation
- ✔ Atrial flutter
- ✔ Transient ischemic attacks (TIAs)
- ✔ Stroke
- ✔ Heart attack
- ✔ Blockages of the arteries
- ✔ After some surgeries
- ✔ Those with disorders of the clotting system

How it Works

Warfarin is a synthetic version of a class of chemicals known as coumarins. These are found in many plants, such as woodruff, lavender and licorice. It was named by combining the acronym for the Wisconsin Alumni Research Foundation (WARF) and the suffix for coumarin (arin). The Foundation provided the original research grants, and it was indeed originally developed as rat poison, but is seldom used as a rat poison today because similar but much more potent forms are now available for that purpose.

Warfarin's anticoagulant effect works because the drug inhibits production of proteins known as "clotting factors." These proteins are produced in the liver and are dependent on an adequate supply of Vitamin K. The clotting factor proteins are the foundation of the "intrinsic" clotting pathway. There are many proteins that work together, and warfarin blocks four of them: Factors VII, IX, X, and II. Creation of these proteins in the liver is dependent on Vitamin K, which can come from dietary sources but can also be created by bacteria in the large intestine. After being absorbed, Vitamin K is stored in the liver. Consequently Vitamin K is the vital regulatory step for the production of the clotting Factors VII, IX, X, and II.

Warfarin blocks the action of Vitamin K within the liver by blocking the absorption sites in the liver needed for the uptake of Vitamin K. With the lowered ability for Vitamin K absorption, there is reduced production of the clotting factors. Consequently, dietary intake of Vitamin K affects the effectiveness of warfarin.

Prescribing Coumadin® (warfarin)

Doctors prescribe Coumadin to patients who are prone to thrombosis and also to prevent them in those who have already formed blood clots. There are numerous conditions that can lead to clot formation, including prosthetic heart valves, atrial fibrillation, deep venous thrombosis and pulmonary embolism. There are also those with inherited problems with clotting factors, like antiphospholipid syndrome and factor five leiden, for whom we prescribe warfarin to prevent clotting. Sometimes the drug is used after myocardial infarction (heart attack) and stroke.

Finding the correct dose of warfarin for patients is complicated by the fact that it interacts with many other over-the-counter and prescription medications, as well as supplements. This interaction can cause Coumadin to be more or less effective. The activity of the drug has to be monitored by frequent blood testing for the international normalized ratio (INR). If the INR is high, the dose is too high. Conversely, if the INR is too low, the medication dose needs to be increased. (We used to use a test, the Prothrombin Time, sometimes called the "Pro Time" or PT, but its accuracy varied between labs. Now results are standardized through the use of the INR.)

Interactions

There are commonly used antibiotics such as erythromycin (Eryc), clarithromycin (Biaxin) and metronidazole (Flagyl) that can markedly increase the effect of Coumadin. In some cases, using antibiotics often changes the amount of the normal bacteria in the intestines and can alter the amount of Vitamin K absorbed into the body.

In addition to other medications, foods that contain higher amounts of Vitamin K also reduce the effectiveness of warfarin. To manage this, there are two basic approaches. One is to try to eat about the same amount of foods that are higher in Vitamin K each day, and the other is to completely eliminate intake of those foods that are high in Vitamin K. The latter strategy is the easier one and the one most recommended by physicians.

Genetics also play a factor in how warfarin is processed in the body. There are tests recently approved by the Food and Drug Administration that can help guide dosing of warfarin.

Adjusting the Dose

It is very important that you always know when will be your next blood test for the INR. It is equally important to know what dose you are taking. It's a good idea to keep a warfarin calendar to help you keep track. Get a small calendar and carry it with you (in your wallet or purse). Write your doses of warfarin in the appropriate days until the next blood test. When you take your dose, circle that day so that you know you have taken it. In the day scheduled for your blood test, write "Get INR" to remind yourself. After the test, if you have not heard from your doctor's office about your results, call them for any new instructions.

The target level of the INR will depend on why you are taking warfarin. In most cases the target range for INR is 2.0-3.0. In some cases, however, the range is higher. Your doctor will set the target based on your particular condition.

Most physicians prefer for their patients to take warfarin in the evening. This is primarily because blood tests are typically taken in the morning, and it will give your doctor time to contact you after your INR is checked. He or she can then change the dose, if needed, before you take your evening medication. There are now home testing kits available and insurance companies are paying for these more and more. Check with your doctor and your insurance company to see if you qualify.

You **must** tell **any** doctor who prescribes medicine for you that you are taking warfarin. If you have any unusual bleeding let your doctor know right away. Call your doctor with any questions or issues earlier rather than later. It's a good idea to have a "Medic Alert" bracelet stating that you are taking warfarin.

Common Side Effects

Rash

On rare occasions warfarin can cause a generalized rash. This has a lacy red pattern and you should call your doctor immediately to discuss this.

Bleeding

The most concerning side effect of warfarin is hemorrhage (bleeding). The risk of severe bleeding is small - on the order of 1 to 2%. In most cases where doctors prescribe warfarin, the benefit will far outweigh the risk. This is why it is so important to take care with your diet as well as other supplements that might interact with the drug.

It may seem difficult and irritating at times for your doctor to have you get your INR level checked, but this is what allows him or her to carefully regulate the drug and reduce the risk of bleeding.

Warfarin Necrosis

A rare complication of warfarin is can be necrosis, or death of skin tissues. This happens more often in people with a deficiency of protein C.

Purple Toe Syndrome

Another rare side effect is known as purple toe syndrome. It generally occurs early after starting the medication -- usually within 3 to 8 weeks. It is thought to be the result of small bits of cholesterol breaking loose from large arteries and flowing into the smaller blood vessels of the feet.

Osteoporosis

Several studies have shown a link between warfarin use and osteoporosis related fractures.

Contraindications

Pregnant women or women who can easily become pregnant should not take warfarin. This is especially true during the first trimester, as it is known to cause deformations of the face and bones of the fetus. During the third trimester there is a high risk of bleeding. There are alternatives such as heparin, however.

Other Interactions

Taking other medications can also increase the risk of bleeding. The most common are antiplatelet drugs such as aspirin, clopidogrel or nonsteroidal anti-inflammatory drugs like ibuprofen (Advil) or naproxyn (Aleve, Naprosyn).

There are many other drug-to-drug interactions, and because of genetic factors the body's processing of the drug can vary widely between patients.

Excessive alcohol use can also affect how warfarin is processed in the liver and elevate the INR. Most physicians will caution patients about the use of alcohol while taking warfarin. Commonly doctors will allow a few drinks after INR is stable.

Foods that are high in Vitamin K have also been reported to interact with warfarin. See the list at the end of this book for a complete list of foods.

Supplements

Warfarin also interacts with many herbs, including (but not limited to):

- ✔ Ginkgo Biloba
- ✔ St. John's Wort
- ✔ American Ginseng
- ✔ Garlic as a supplement (not fresh garlic)

Vitamin K Dosage

I get the question all the time about how much Vitamin K is right for folks taking Coumadin® (warfarin). Unfortunately, there's no perfect study to guide just how much Vitamin K is too much for those taking Coumadin. Most physicians recommend limiting foods that contain very high or even moderate amounts of Vitamin K. At the same time, there's never been a recommendation to severely limit Vitamin K intake.

The Recommended Daily Allowance (RDA) for Vitamin K is 80 micrograms (mcg) for males and 70 mcg for females. The majority of ingredients contain small amounts - in the under 15 mcg range - so keeping an eye on foods that contain more than 20 - 25 mcg per serving is a good rule of thumb.

Avoiding **all** Vitamin K might be just as much of a problem as getting too much, however. Studies have clearly shown that eating foods that are higher in Vitamin K will have an effect on the effectiveness of Coumadin and the INR. Most people who either take warfarin themselves or those who help patients manage their anti-coagulation know this, but there is some research now that shows eating too little Vitamin K can have the same effect.

So what to do? How much is too much? How little is too little? It appears, from what research we have, that in those folks who were taking Coumadin, 29 mcg was too little and 76 mcg just right to keep their INR stable.

While it's not a perfect way to look at the issue of how much is too much Vitamin K in the diet for warfarin users, another study showed an effect on the INR in those taking 150 - 200 mcg per day in Vitamin K supplements. These are the levels found in Vitamin K rich foods such as spinach, collard greens and broccoli.

For the number of folks who use this medication and the fact that there's no great replacement on the horizon, it is a shame that a large study has not been done to help answer this question more clearly. For the time being, we have to be content with the small studies that point toward an optimum near the RDA guidelines for Vitamin K.

Pictures of Coumadin® (warfarin) tablets

You can find pictures of warfarin pills on the Dr. Gourmet web site at this address:
www.drgourmet.com/warfarin/tablets

How to Use This Diet

The first step is to determine your target weight. Using the appropriate table (Men or Women) on the next page, find your height in the left column. Then read across the row for your Ideal Body Weight. This is an estimated target weight based on CDC and World Health Organization guidelines. There can be other factors in determining your goal weight, so it's important to check with your physician about what is a good target for you.

After you have identified an Ideal Body Weight, there is an estimate for the total caloric intake needed for weight loss (to get to that weight) as well as a maintenance diet (to maintain that weight once you've achieved your goal).
The table below translates your total daily caloric intake into the number of servings of each recipe you should be eating.

Calories	● Breakfast	▲ Lunch	■ Dinner	Extras
1000	●	▲	■	
1200	●	▲ ▲	■	
1500	● ●	▲ ▲	■	
1800	● ●	▲ ▲	■ ■	
2000	● ●	▲ ▲	■ ■	

Female

Height (in inches)	Ideal Body Weight	For weight Loss	Maintenance
60	105	1000	1200
61	110	1000	1200
62	115	1000	1200
63	120	1000	1200
64	125	1200	1500
65	130	1200	1500
66	135	1200	1500
67	140	1200	1500
68	145	1200	1500
69	150	1500	1800
70	155	1500	1800
71	160	1500	1800
72	165	1500	1800

Male

Height (in inches)	Ideal Body Weight	For weight Loss	Maintenance
60	106	1000	1200
61	112	1000	1200
62	118	1000	1200
63	124	1000	1200
64	130	1200	1500
65	136	1200	1500
66	142	1200	1500
67	148	1200	1500
68	154	1200	1800
69	160	1200	1800
70	166	1500	1800
71	172	1500	1800
72	178	1500	2000
73	184	1500	2000
74	190	1500	2000
75	196	1500	2000
76	202	1500	2000

More About the Recipes

Recipes and menus have been labeled with a circle, triangle or square so that you can swap them easily in case you're allergic to a particular food.

● The Circle recipes are for breakfast.

▲ Triangle recipes are for lunch.

■ Squares are for dinner recipes or menus. Often a side dish is recommended with the main course for dinner, and that is included in the square (your serving). Side dishes, or Extras, have no shapes assigned for this reason.

One square is equivalent to two triangles. (That is, one serving of a dinner menu or meal is equivalent to two lunch servings.)

■ = ▲ ▲

Each individual recipe is labeled with the number of servings it makes inside each shape. For instance, this square shows you that the recipe will serve 2:

■

Each recipe has the approximate time next to it. Here is a dinner recipe that will take about 45 minutes to prepare and will serve two:

2 **45 min.**

Menus that take more than 30 minutes will usually have leftovers or are for special occasion meals.

The Rules

1. If you don't like a particular food and want to substitute one recipe for another, be sure to choose a recipe with the same number of servings (and time value). For instance, you could have Candied Carrots with your Creamy Mac and Cheese instead of the Herbed Zucchini. Or you could trade Oven Fried Chicken for the Thai Coconut Shrimp.

2. Shopping lists are provided for you, with all the ingredients needed for each week's menus. The plan is designed to run Sunday through Saturday so that you can shop on Saturday, although you can start any day you wish and adjust the menu days accordingly.

3. Take some time to read through the recipes and the plan on Saturday before going to the store. There may be ingredients or techniques that you are not familiar with, or you may need to marinate a recipe the night before it is to be served. Likewise, there are equipment lists for each week that can help you to make sure that you have all the gear needed.

4. The plan does call for making some food on Sunday afternoon or evening to eat during the week (those are usually recipes that take more than 30 minutes).

Breakfast and lunch, when not specified in the weekly menu, are outlined in the Breakfast and Lunch Guidelines with options for menus for both meals.

6. There are meals scheduled for eating out. The rule is that you can order **any entree that doesn't contain ingredients high in vitamin K on the menu and eat half of it.** The other half is eaten the following day for lunch.

7. Lastly, there is **no between meal snacking.** Patients have told me that the first week or two can be a little more difficult, so you can have a piece of fruit for a snack if you really need one.

A word or two about what to drink

For the first six weeks I recommend that you don't drink any alcohol that is not on the diet. Depending on your health condition your doctor may not want you to drink alcohol at all and you should check with him or her about this before having any alcoholic beverages. You will find that I feel alcohol can be good for you, but at first you should avoid it primarily due to the calories in wine, beer or mixed drinks. There are a few meals that call for a beer or margarita and this is part of the plan. After you have reached your maintenance weight, drink in moderation, remembering that all alcohol has calories.

Coffee and tea are not bad for you, in my opinion, but many of us do drink too much and cutting back may be something you want to think about. If you use sugar, change to Splenda® or another non-calorie product. If you use cream or half and half, switch to 2% milk. As far as other liquids go, you may drink pretty much anything that doesn't have calories. I am not much of a fan of sodas (diet or regular) but if you are going to have them, drink only calorie free products. I do feel that you would be better off to eliminate them from your life and drink water.

Water is great for you and you almost can't drink too much. The idea that it can fill you up and help you eat less may actually be true. Either way, this is good stuff. For many of us it is an acquired taste after having been saturated with so many sodas and sugary drinks. Work on drinking less soda and more water.

Breakfast Guidelines

Option No. 1

Cereal with Milk (or Yogurt) and a piece of Fruit

Cereals should have about 100 - 150 calories in a serving. 1/2 cup of skim or 1% milk is ideal. Using a half cup of non-fat yogurt is even better.

Cereal	Amount per serving	Comment
Cheerios	1 cup (30 grams)	Multi-grain are best!
Kellogg's All-Bran Bran Buds	1/2 cup (45 grams)	
Kellogg's All-Bran Extra Fiber	1 cup	
Kellogg's All-Bran Original	1 cup	
Kellogg's Special K	1 cup (30 grams)	
Kellogg's Special K with Red Berries	1 cup (31 grams)	
Bite Size Shredded Wheat	1 cup (52 grams)	Not frosted
Raisin Bran	1 cup	
Total Whole Grain	1 cup	
Total Raisin Bran	1 cup	
Kashi Cinnamon Harvest	1 cup	
Kashi GoLEAN	1 cup (53 grams)	
Oatmeal	1/4 cup	(before cooking)
Cream of Wheat	1/4 cup	(before cooking)

A word about Cereal Bars:

Cereal bars are for emergencies only. Eating a granola bar for breakfast is not a good substitute. Many of them have a lot of added calories (usually as sugar).

Option No. 2

Breads and Protein and a piece of Fruit

Breads should be served with a protein. Select one from the bread choices, a topping for your bread and one choice from the protein list.

Breads	Amount	Comment
Slice of Whole Wheat Toast	One	Choose whole grain breads
Bagel	1/2 large bagel	
Whole wheat English Muffin	1 whole muffin	
Muffin from recipe @ drgourmet.com	One	
Toppings & Spreads for Breads	**Amount**	**Comment**
Choose one only Take Control Light Spread	2 tsp.	
Promise Buttery Spread Light	2 tsp.	
Smart Balance Light Buttery Spread	2 tsp.	(Omega Plus is better)
Preserves or Jam	2 tsp.	Look for "low sugar"
Reduced-fat Cream Cheese	2 tsp.	The "light" cream cheese is best for spreading. I don't much like the "fat free" version and use it mostly in baking
Take Control Light Spread and Syrup or honey	2 tsp. and 1 Tbsp.	Topping for pancakes or French Toast
Protein	**Amount**	**Comment**
1 Large Egg	One	Cook in as little fat as possible
Peanut Butter	2 Tbsp.	Use instead of other spreads
Low-fat cheese	1/2 ounce	
2%, 1% or Skim Milk	1/2 cup	
Non-fat Yogurt	1 cup	Choose yogurt with no added sugar

Lunch Guidelines

Sandwiches, defined:

- **Whole Sandwich** = 2 lunch servings (two triangles)

  2 slices whole wheat bread with 2 ounces lean meat OR 2 ounces reduced-fat cheese

- **Half Sandwich** = 1 lunch serving (one triangle)

  1 slice whole wheat bread with 1 ounce lean meat OR 1 ounce reduced-fat cheese

Meat & Cheese Choices

Reduced-fat Swiss

Reduced-fat Cheddar

Reduced-fat Monterey Jack

Goat Cheese

Lean Ham slices

Lean Turkey slices

2 Tbsp. Peanut Butter

Sandwich extras (put on as much as you like):

Sliced tomato

Sliced peppers

Onions

Spreads

Hellman's Extra Light Mayonnaise: 1 Tbsp.

Any Coarse Ground Mustard: 1 Tbsp.

Dijon Style Mustard: 1 Tbsp.

Your Favorite Chutney: 1 Tbsp.

Roasted Garlic: 2 cloves

Tapenade: 1 Tbsp.

Leftovers

Remember, a lunch serving is one-half of a leftover dinner serving.

Weekly Meal Plans

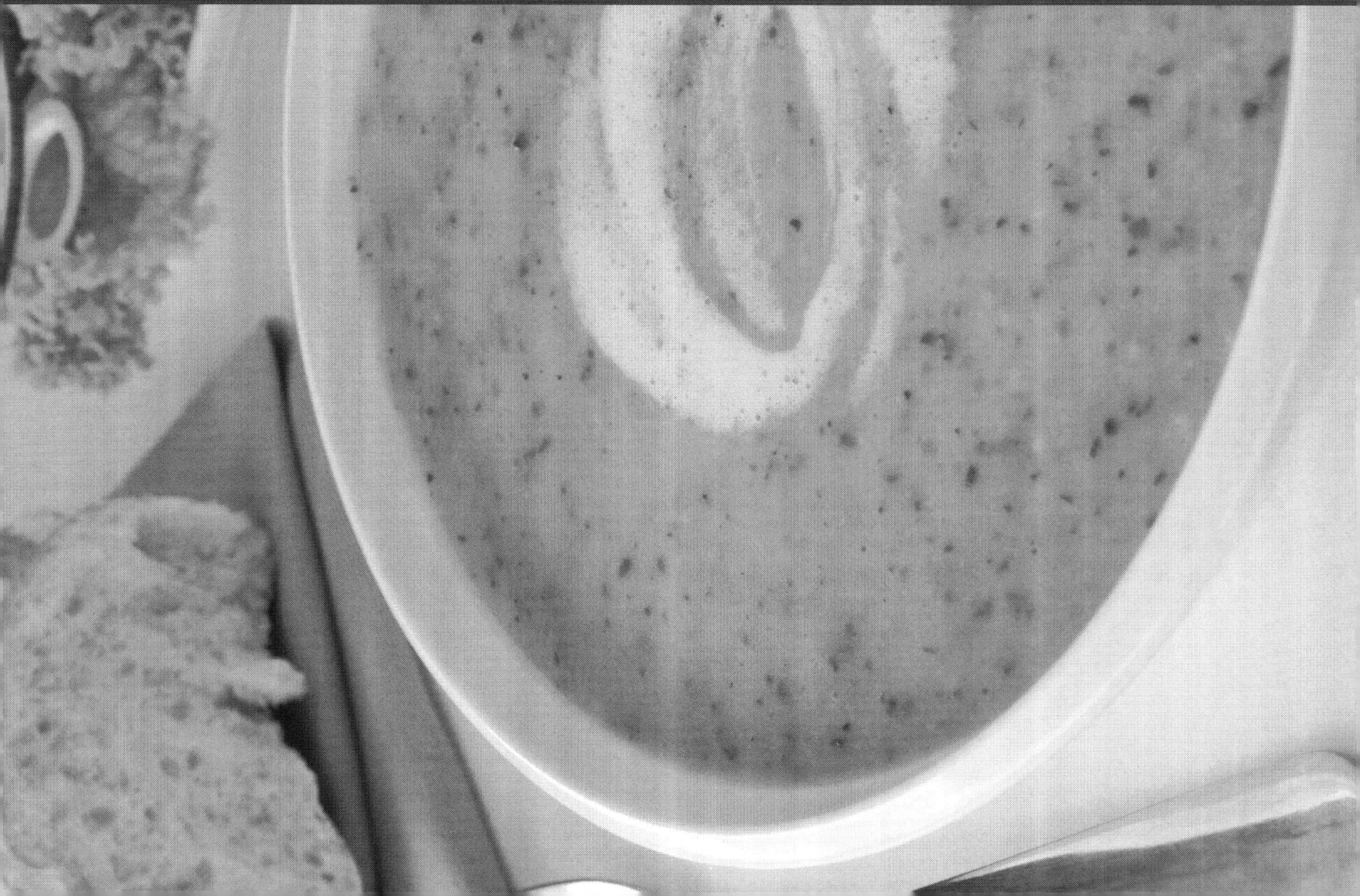

Week 1 Meal Plan				
	● Breakfast	▲ Lunch	■ Dinner	To Do
Sunday	1 serving Apple Pancake with 1 Tbsp. Take Control Spread Light and 1 Tbsp. Maple Syrup, Juice	1 serving Curried Chicken Salad & one 2 oz. pita bread, Fruit	Pizza with Tomato, Basil and Roasted Garlic	Make Blueberry Muffins, Make Whole Wheat Pizza Dough Roast Garlic
Monday	Blueberry Muffin, Fruit	1 serving Curried Chicken Salad & one 2 oz. pita bread, Fruit	Creamy Macaroni & Cheese, Candied Carrots	1/2 serving Apple Pancake for snack
Tuesday	Blueberry Muffin, Fruit	1/2 serving Creamy Macaroni & Cheese, Fruit,	Thai Coconut Shrimp Thai Peanut Sauce, Coconut Rice, Thai Cucumber Salad	1/2 serving Apple Pancake for snack
Wednesday	Bagel with 1 oz. Low-fat cream cheese, Fruit	1/2 serving Creamy Macaroni & Cheese, Fruit	Salmon with Parmesan Crust, Jasmine Rice, Herbed Zucchini	
Thursday	Blueberry Muffin, Fruit	2 oz. Thai Coconut Shrimp & 1 slice bread with peanut sauce, Thai Cucumber Salad (Sandwich)	Lentil and Black Bean Salad, 1 ounce whole wheat roll spread with Roasted Garlic	
Friday	Cereal with 1/2 cup 1% milk, Fruit	2 oz. Thai Coconut Shrimp & 1 slice bread with peanut sauce, Cucumber Salad (Sandwich)	Fettuccine Alfredo, Green Beans with Walnut Vinaigrette	Make only a half recipe of Green Bean Salad
Saturday	Scrambled Eggs, Slice Toast with 1 Tbsp. Take Control Spread Light or 1 Tbsp. Jam	1/2 serving Lentil and Black Bean Salad, 1/2 serving Leftover Green Beans with Walnut Vinaigrette	London Broil with Mushrooms Sautéed in Cognac, Roasted Garlic Mashed Potatoes, Green Beans with Red Onion	Make only a half recipe of Green Beans with Red Onion

Week 1 Grocery List

Produce

2 lbs. granny smith apples
1 bunch Green Onions
1 small bunch Celery
1 Red Bell Pepper
1 medium Tomato
1 small bunch Fresh Basil
1/2 cup Blueberries
3 heads Garlic
3 large Shallots
2 Limes
1 small piece Fresh Ginger Root
1 medium bunch Thai Basil
(Sweet Basil will do)
2 small Red Onions
2 large Cucumbers
1 small bunch Cilantro Leaves
8 oz. Zucchini
Green Beans
1 Lemon
1 1/4 lbs. Fresh Green Beans
1 lb. Yukon Gold Potatoes
1 lb. fresh Crimini Mushrooms
1 small bunch Fresh Thyme
16 Servings Fruit
8 oz. peeled Baby Carrots
1 Tbl. parsley

Dairy

1 stick Unsalted Butter
6 large eggs
1 qt. Non-fat Buttermilk
1 oz. per serving Fresh Mozzarella
2 oz. Parmigiano-Reggiano
1/2 cup Egg Substitute
2 Tbsp. Non-fat Yogurt
1 quart 1% Milk
5 oz. Low-fat Extra-sharp Cheddar Cheese
1 quart 2% Milk
1 ounce Semi-soft Goat Cheese
Reduced-fat Cream Cheese
1 tub Promise Buttery Spread or Smart Balance Spread
1 tub Take Control Light spread

Meat/Fish

1 - 4 ounce chicken breasts
1 lb. Large Shrimp
2 – 4 oz. Salmon Filets
1 lb. Lean London Broil

Bakery

2 oz. fresh Sourdough Bread
2 - 1 oz. Whole Wheat Rolls

Pantry Items

Splenda
Curry Powder
Ground Cinnamon
Granulated Sugar
Pure Vanilla Extract
Salt
Baking Powder & Baking Soda
Cornstarch
Black Pepper
Red Pepper Flakes
Pure Walnut Extract
1 bag All-purpose Flour
Low-fat Mayonnaise
Slivered Almonds
Chutney
2 Tbsp. Golden Raisins
1 tsp. Dry Active Yeast
Extra Virgin Olive Oil
1 can Spray Olive Oil
Grapeseed Oil
1 lb. Whole Wheat Fettuccine
Rice Vinegar
Balsamic Vinegar
White Wine Vinegar
1/2 lb. Penne Pasta
1 can Low-fat Coconut Milk
Low-sodium Soy Sauce
Hoisin Sauce
Pure Maple Syrup
Reduced-fat Peanut Butter
Non-fat Chicken Stock
1 can Non-fat Beef Stock
Tabasco Sauce
Jasmine Rice
1 - 15 oz. can no-salt added Black Beans
Red Lentils
Green Lentils
Dijon Mustard
Low-fat Croutons
Cognac or Brandy or Bourbon

Equipment

Medium Cast Iron Skillet
Medium Mixing Bowl
Pizza Stone
Large Spatula
Muffin Papers
Muffin Tin
Garlic Roaster or Medium Sauce Pan with Lid
Large Non-stick Skillet or Grill Pan
Wooden Skewers
Medium Whisk
Small Sauté Pan

Week 2 Meal Plan				
	● Breakfast	▲ Lunch	■ Dinner	To Do
Sunday	Blueberry Buttermilk Pancakes with 1 Tbsp. Take Control Spread Light and 1 Tbsp. Maple Syrup, Juice	1 oz. 2% Swiss Cheese with 1/2 of the cognac and mushrooms on 1 slice whole grain bread (Sandwich)	Butternut Squash Risotto	Make Roasted Eggplant Soup (recipe at www. DrGourmet.com/ recipes/soup)
Monday	Blueberry Muffin, Fruit	1 serving Eggplant Soup with 1 oz. whole wheat roll spread with Roasted Garlic, Fruit	Philly Cheese Steak	
Tuesday	Cereal with 1/2 cup 1% milk, Fruit	1/2 serving Butternut Squash Risotto, Fruit	Seared Tuna Steak with Sake-Wasabi Sauce, Brown Rice	
Wednesday	Blueberry Muffin, Fruit	1 serving Eggplant Soup with 1 oz. whole wheat roll spread with Roasted Garlic, Fruit	Sea Bass with White Beans and Tomato Vinaigrette	
Thursday	Blueberry Muffin, Fruit	1/2 serving Butternut Squash Risotto, Fruit	Minestrone, 1 oz. whole wheat roll with 1 oz. cheese, Fruit	
Friday	Bagel with 1 oz. Low-fat cream cheese, Fruit	1 serving Eggplant Soup with 1 oz. whole wheat roll spread with Roasted Garlic, Fruit	Oven Fried Fish, (recipe at www.DrGourmet.com/ recipes/maincourse/fish French Fries Cocktail Sauce, Fruit	Make half the recipe of the French Fries
Saturday	Cereal with 1/2 cup 1% milk, Fruit	Minestrone, Fruit	2 oz. Pasta with Tomato Sauce topped with 1/2 oz. Parmigiano-Reggiano, Herbed Zucchini	Make the Tomato Sauce, puree the leftover sauce and freeze 2 1/2 cups Make a half of a recipe of the Herbed Zucchini

Week 2 Grocery List

Produce

1 – 2 lb. Butternut Squash
2 large Leeks
◆ 2 medium Red Onion
1/2 lb. Plum Tomatoes
1 1/2 lbs. Eggplant
◆ 2 bulbs Garlic
◆ 6 medium Onions
◆ 1 Lime
◆ 1 large Shallot
12 Tomatoes
1 small Zucchini
1 lb. Carrot
1/2 lb. Parsnips
◆ 3 ribs Celery
1 1/2 lbs. Red Potatoes
◆ 2 Tbsp. Lemon Juice
1/2 lb. Russet Potatoes
22 servings Fruit

Dairy

◆ 2/3 cup Non-fat Buttermilk
◆ 1/4 cup Egg Substitute
◆ Take Control Light Margarine
◆ 3 oz. Parmigiano-Reggiano
◆ 2 large eggs
1/2 oz. Low-fat Swiss Cheese (per serving)
◆ 3 Tbsp. Unsalted Butter
◆ 2 cups 1% Milk
2 oz. Low-fat Cheddar Cheese

Meat/Fish

2 – 4 oz. Tuna Steaks
2 – 4 oz. filets Sea Bass
4 - 4 oz. Cod Filets

Bakery

1 Mini-Baguette (per serving)
2 - 1 oz. Whole Wheat Rolls

Pantry Items

◆ All-purpose Flour
◆ Splenda
◆ Baking Powder
◆ Pure Vanilla Extract
◆ Pure Maple Syrup
◆ Spray Olive Oil
◆ Extra Virgin Olive Oil
1 cup Arborio Rice
◆ 9 cups Non-fat Chicken Stock
1/4 cup Dry Sherry
◆ Salt
◆ Black Pepper
Ground Paprika
Dried Thyme
1/2 cups White Wine
1 Tbsp. Non-fat Mayonnaise
◆ Low-sodium Soy Sauce
Sake
◆ Honey
Wasabi Paste
Dark Sesame Oil
2/3 cup Brown Rice
1 oz. Dried Wild Mushroom (like Porcini)
1 - 15 ounce can White Beans
◆ 1/4 tsp. Dried Oregano
1 lb. Great Northern Beans
Bay Leaves
◆ ounces Plain Melba Toast
◆ 1 Tbsp. Dijon Mustard
3 Tbsp. Prepared Horseradish
3/4 Tbsp. no salt added Ketchup
Tabasco Sauce
4 – 28 oz. cans Whole Peeled Tomatoes or 4 lbs. fresh Tomatoes
4 ounces pasta of your choice (preferably whole wheat)
Fresh Herbs of your choice

Equipment

◆ Non-stick Griddle
◆ Large Stock Pot
Medium Roasting Pan
◆ Stick Blender

◆ indicates previously purchased - check pantry first

Week 3 Meal Plan				
	● Breakfast	▲ Lunch	■ Dinner	To Do
Sunday	Jean's French Toast with 1 Tbsp. Take Control Spread Light and 1 Tbsp. Maple Syrup, Juice	1/2 Sandwich using 1/2 serving leftover Oven Fried Fish and Cocktail Sauce, Fruit	Beef Stew	Make Orange Blueberry Scones Make Beef Stew
Monday	Scone, Fruit	Minestrone, Fruit	Pepperoni Pizza	Make Pizza Dough in time for dinner
Tuesday	Scone, Fruit	1/2 serving Beef Stew	Linguine with Shrimp in Vodka Cream using 1 medium diced zucchini per serving instead of the asparagus	Thaw Tomato Sauce in advance for the Linguine recipe (make the recipe using only half of the shrimp)
Wednesday	Scone, Fruit	Minestrone, Fruit	Fettuccini with Dill Pesto and Shrimp	Make Dill Pesto Use zucchini instead of the white asparagus in the fettuccini recipe
Thursday	Cereal with half cup 1% milk, Fruit	1/2 serving Linguine and pasta (no Shrimp)	Mediterranean Chicken Salad	
Friday	Cereal with half cup 1% milk, Fruit	1/2 Sandwich on whole grain bread using 1/2 serving leftover Mediterranean Chicken Salad	Plzza with Dill Pesto and Potato	Make Pizza Dough in time for dinner Thaw Tomato Sauce for the Baked Penne
Saturday	Zucchini and Chevre Frittata with 1 Slice Toast with 1 Tbsp. Take Control Spread Light or 1 Tbsp. Jam	1/2 Sandwich on whole grain bread using 1/2 serving leftover Mediterranean Chicken Salad	Baked Penne (use thawed tomato sauce)	Freeze remaining Baked Penne in single serving Ziplock bags

Week 3 Grocery List

Produce

25 Pearl Onions
1/2 lb. Button Mushrooms
1 lb. Carrots
2 lbs. Red Potatoes
1 Tbsp Lemon Juice
1 lb. Carrots
1 1/2 lbs. Red Potatoes
1 Orange
1/4 cup Blueberries
16 spears large Asparagus
4 large Shallots
1 small bunch Fresh Basil
◆ 1 bulb Garlic
1 bunch fresh Dill
4 medium Zucchini
◆ 8 ounces Grape Tomatoes
◆ 12 Black Olives
8 leaves fresh Basil
◆ 2 Red Onions
2 Yellow Peppers
3 Red Peppers
1 lb. Eggplant
1 small bunch Fresh Oregano
16 servings Fresh Fruit

Dairy

◆ 3/4 cup Egg Substitute
◆ 1 Egg
◆ Take Control Light Margarine
◆ 5 Tbsp. Unsalted Butter
1 cup Fat-free Sour Cream
1 3/4 cup 2% Milk
◆ 1 ounce Goat Cheese
◆ 1 cup Non-fat Buttermilk
2 oz. Part-skim Milk Mozzarella
◆ 3 oz. Parmigiano-Reggiano
◆ 1 oz. Fresh Mozzarella
3 oz. Fontina Cheese
1 oz. Pecorino-Romano Cheese

Meat/Fish

1 1/2 lbs. Flank Steak
Hormel Low-salt Turkey Pepperoni
1 lb. Large Shrimp
1 lb. Boneless Chicken Breasts

Bakery

4 slices fresh Sourdough Bread
2 - 1 oz. Whole Wheat Rolls

Pantry Items

◆ Splenda
Ground Nutmeg
◆ Pure Vanilla Extract
◆ Salt
◆ Pure Maple Syrup
1 Tbsp Low Sodium Worcestershire Sauce
◆ Ground Allspice
◆ 2 Bay Leaves
1 lb. box Penne Pasta
◆ Black Pepper
◆ 4 cups All Purpose Flour
1/4 cup Light Brown Sugar
◆ Baking Powder
1/2 cup Sun Dried Tomatoes
1/2 cup Vodka
8 ounces Linguine
2 Tbsp. Pine Nuts
◆ 4 ounces Fettuccine
◆ Extra Virgin Olive Oil
◆ Spray Olive Oil
◆ 2 Tbsp. Balsamic Vinegar
◆ 1 Tbsp. Honey

Equipment

◆ Non-stick Griddle
◆ Medium Whisk
Medium Mixing Bowl
◆ Large Stock Pot
◆ Pizza Stone
◆ Large Spatula
◆ Large Non-stick Skillet
Blender or Mini Chopper
1 - 12 inch Oblong Pyrex Dish

◆ indicates previously purchased - check pantry first

Week 4

Week 4 Meal Plan				
	● Breakfast	▲ Lunch	■ Dinner	To Do
Sunday	Blueberry Blue Cornmeal Pancakes, 1 Tbsp. Take Control Spread Light, 1 Tbsp. Maple Syrup	1/2 serving Baked Penne	Meatloaf, Plain Mashed Potatoes, Roasted Beets	Make Pumpkin Nut Muffins Make beets without parsley
Monday	Pumpkin Muffin, Fruit	1/2 Sandwich on whole grain bread using 1/2 serving leftover Meatloaf, Fruit	Roasted Salmon with Red Thai Curry, Coconut Rice, 1/2 serving Roasted Acorn Squash	
Tuesday	Bagel / 1 Tbsp. Light Cream Cheese / Fruit	1/2 Sandwich on whole grain bread using 1/2 serving leftover Meatloaf, Fruit	Indian Shrimp Curry, Coconut Rice, 1/2 serving leftover Roasted Acorn Squash	
Wednesday	Pumpkin Muffin, Fruit	1/2 serving Indian Shrimp Curry & 1/2 serving Coconut Rice	Mushroom Risotto	
Thursday	Cereal / half cup 1% milk / Fruit	Mushroom Risotto	Roasted Salmon with Corn Relish (leave out the parsley)	
Friday	Pumpkin Muffin, Fruit	1/2 serving Indian Shrimp Curry & 1/2 serving Coconut Rice	Corn Quesadillas, Jicama Salad, 1 twelve oz. beer or a 5 ounce glass of wine	(check with your doctor about alcohol use)
Saturday	Bagel with 1 oz. Light Cream Cheese, 1 oz. Smoked Salmon, Fruit	1/2 serving Baked Penne	Barbecue Chicken, Roasted Corn, Parmesan Squash	

Week 4 Grocery List

Produce

2 Tbsp. fresh Blueberries (per serving)
◆ 6 cloves Garlic
◆ 2 1/2 medium White Onion
1/2 lb. Yukon Gold Potatoes
2 large Yellow Squash
1 Avocado
◆ 1 small bunch Fresh Cilantro
1 small Tomato
◆ 5 fresh Limes
◆ 1 medium Red Onion
1 Acorn Squash
2 oz. Wild Type Mushrooms
◆ 1 small bunch Fresh Basil
1 medium Tomatoe
1 Red Bell Pepper
1/2 lb. Shiitaki Mushrooms
1 Poblano Chili
◆ 1 1/2 tsp. Fresh Thyme
4 ears Yellow or White Corn
◆ 3 Green Onions
◆ 1 small Shallot
1 medium Jicama
1 Medium Beet
14 Servings Fruit

Dairy

◆ 1 cup Non-fat Buttermilk
3/4 cup Egg Substitute
◆ Take Control Light Margarine
Reduced-fat Monterey Jack Cheese
◆ 4 tsp. Unsalted Butter
◆ 1 cup 2% milk
◆ 2 1/2 ounces Parmigiano-Reggiano
◆ Light Cream Cheese

Meat/Fish

4 – 4 oz. Salmon Filets
1 lb. Large Shrimp
1 – 4 oz. chicken breast, thigh or drumstick (per serving)
1 lb. Extra Lean Ground Beef

Bakery

4 oz. Sourdough Bread (for bread crumbs)

Pantry Items

1/2 cup Blue Cornmeal
1/4 cup Whole Wheat Flour
◆ 1 1/2 cups Splenda
◆ Baking Powder
◆ Salt
◆ Pure Vanilla Extract
◆ Pure Maple Syrup
◆ Dried Oregano & Basil
◆ Dried Rosemary & Thyme
3/4 cup Tomato Sauce (may use from previously frozen)
◆ Chili Powder
1/2 Tsp. Hot Red Bean Paste
◆ 1 cup Reduced-fat Coconut Milk
2 Tbsp. Sake or Dry White Wine
◆ 1 tsp. Sesame Oil
◆ 1 cup All Purpose Flour
◆ Baking Powder
◆ Baking Soda
◆ Ground Nutmeg
◆ Ground Allspice
◆ Ground Cinnamon
◆ 2 Tbsp. Golden Raisins
◆ 1 can Canned Pumpkin
◆ 1 tsp. Granulated Sugar
◆ Extra Virgin Olive Oil
◆ Cornstarch
◆ Curry Powder
◆ Honey
◆ 1 cup Low-fat Unsweetened Coconut Milk
◆ 1 cup Arborio Rice
◆ 2/3 cup White Wine
◆ Ground Paprika
◆ 2 tsp. Brown Sugar
◆ Ground Cumin
◆ 4 tsp. Grapeseed Oil

Equipment

◆ Non-stick Griddle
◆ Medium Whisk
◆ Muffin Tin
◆ Muffin Papers
◆ Non-stick Griddle

◆ indicates previously purchased - check pantry first

Week 5 Meal Plan				
	● Breakfast	▲ Lunch	■ Dinner	To Do
Sunday	Four Grain Pancakes with 2 tsp. Take Control Light Spread and 1 Tbsp. Maple Syrup	1 ounce Barbecue chicken on 1 slice bread (Sandwich), Fruit	Ginger Cilantro Flank Steak, Purple Sticky Rice, Thai Cucumber Salad	Make Jerk Seasoning
Monday	Pumpkin Nut Muffin, Fruit	1 ounce Barbecue chicken on 1 slice bread (Sandwich), Fruit	3 oz. Flank Steak on Jicama Salad with Melon Salsa	Make Melon Salsa
Tuesday	Cereal with 1/2 cup 1% milk, Fruit	1 oz. Flank Steak on 1 slice bread (Sandwich)	Jerk Shrimp, Coconut Rice, Melon Salsa	
Wednesday	Pumpkin Nut Muffin, Fruit	2 ounces Jerk Shrimp on 1 slice bread (Sandwich)	Chicken with Tarragon Mustard Cream, Roasted Garlic Mashed Potatoes, Green Beans with Red Onions	
Thursday	Pumpkin Nut Muffin, Fruit	2 oz. Jerk Shrimp on 1 slice bread (Sandwich)	Pizza with Thai Peanut Sauce and Scallop	Make Pizza Dough in time for dinner Marinate Lamb Kabobs (do not use parsley in the marinade for the lamb)
Friday	Bagel, 1 Tbsp. Light Cream Cheese, Fruit	1/2 serving Baked Penne	Lamb Kabobs, Couscous	Thaw Tomato Sauce for the Gnocchi
Saturday	Tortilla, Fruit	1/2 serving Baked Penne	Gnocchi with Tomato Sauce and 1/2 oz. grated Parmigiano-Reggiano	

Week 5 Grocery List

Produce

1 - 2 inch piece Ginger Root
1 small bunch Cilantro Leaves
1 small Red Bell Pepper
◆ 2 Limes
6 oz. Cantaloupe
4 oz. Honeydew
1 small Green Bell Pepper
1 small bunch Fresh Sage
1 small bunch Fresh Chives
7 medium Red Potatoes
6 large Shiitake Mushrooms
2 medium White Onions
◆ 1 Green Onion
1 small bunch Fresh Basil
1 small bunch Fresh Oregano
1 small Jalapeno Pepper
10 oz. Yukon Gold Potatoes
1 Medium Red Onion
1 large Leek
1/2 cup Mung Bean Sprouts
1/2 lb. Green Beans
16 servings Fruit

Dairy

◆ 1 cup Non-fat Buttermilk
◆ 3/4 cup 2% Milk
◆ 2 Large Eggs
◆ 2 tsp. Take Control Light Spread
◆ 1 tsp. Unsalted Butter
◆ 2 oz. Goat Cheese
◆ 1 Tbsp. Egg Substitute
◆ 1 oz. grated Parmigiano-Reggiano
◆ Light Cream Cheese
◆ 2 Tbsp. Promise Buttery Spread or Smart Balance Spread

Meat/Fish

1 lb. Flank Steak
8 oz. Large Shrimp
2 – 4 ounce Boneless Skinless Chicken Breasts
6 Sea Scallops
8 oz. Lean Lamb Shoulder

Bakery

10 slices Whole Grain Bread
2 Bagels

Pantry Items

◆ 1/4 cup Reduced-fat Coconut Milk
◆ Cornstarch
◆ Splenda
2 Tbsp. Unsalted Dry Roasted Peanuts
◆ Salt
1 tsp. Baking Powder
◆ Low-sodium Soy Sauce
◆ Rice Vinegar
◆ Dark Sesame Oil
◆ 6 Tbsp. Non-fat Chicken Stock
◆ 1/2 Tsp. Hot Red Bean Paste
1 small Dried Chipotle
Black Peppercorns
Onion Powder
◆ Ground Allspice & Cinnamon
◆ Ground Cumin & Nutmeg
Coriander Seed
Ground Ginger
◆ Whole Wheat Flour
◆ All-purpose Flour
◆ Yellow Corn Meal
◆ 6 Tbsp. Oatmeal
◆ Chili Powder
◆ Extra Virgin Olive Oil
◆ Coarse Ground Mustard
Dried Tarragon
◆ Pure Maple Syrup
◆ Dry Sherry
1 cup Couscous
1/2 cup Dried Currants
Red Pepper Flakes
Reduced-fat Peanut Butter
2 tsp. Tabasco Sauce
◆ 1 tsp. Fresh Thyme
Dried Thyme
◆ Light Brown Sugar
Whole Cloves
◆ Grapeseed Oil

Equipment

◆ Non-stick Grill Pan
Large Slotted Spoon
Skewers

◆ indicates previously purchased - check pantry first

Week 6 Meal Plan				
	● Breakfast	▲ Lunch	■ Dinner	To Do
Sunday	Orange French Toast with 2 tsp. Take Control Spread and 1 Tbsp. Orange Honey	1/2 Serving leftover Gnocchi	Halibut with Seven Spice Powder, Rice and Lentil Pilaf	Marinate Mojo Pork Tenderloin Make Muffin of your choice
Monday	Muffin, Fruit	Leftover Tortilla, Fruit	Mojo Pork Tenderloin Melon Salsa, Dirty Rice	
Tuesday	1/2 Bagel with 1 ounce Light cream cheese, Fruit	2 oz. Pork tenderloin on 1 slice bread with salsa (Sandwich), Fruit	Curried Sea Scallops, Coconut Rice, Herbed Zucchini	
Wednesday	Cereal with 1/2 cup 1% milk, Fruit	2 oz. Pork tenderloin on 1 slice bread with salsa (Sandwich), Fruit	Tomato Saffron Risotto with Salmon	
Thursday	Cereal with 1/2 cup 1% milk, Fruit	1/2 serving Tomato Saffron Risotto with Salmon, Fruit	Oven Fried Chicken, Roast Corn, Roasted Beets	
Friday	Muffin, Fruit	1/2 serving Tomato Saffron Risotto with Salmon, Fruit	Eat Out (fowl)	
Saturday	Four Grain Pancakes with 2 tsp. Take Control Light Spread and 1 Tbsp. Maple Syrup	1/2 serving Oven Fried Chicken on 1 slice bread (Sandwich)	Chili Rellenos	

Week 6 Grocery List

Produce

3 Navel Oranges
2 medium Shallots
1 Tbsp. All-purpose Flour
◆ 1 Lime
2 medium Beets
◆ 1 Tbsp. Fresh Oregano
◆ 1 bulb Garlic
2 ears Yellow Corn
◆ 1 small bunch Fresh Cilantro
◆ 1/2 Red Bell Pepper
◆ 1/2 Yellow Bell Pepper
◆ 1/2 Green Bell Pepper
1 lb. Tomatoes
1 small Cucumber
◆ 1 Lemon (use zest for Curried Sea Scallops)
◆ 3 medium White Onions
4 small Zucchini
4 medium Poblano Peppers
◆ Whole Wheat Flour
◆ All-purpose Flour
◆ Yellow Corn Meal
◆ 6 Tbsp. Oatmeal
1 large Leek
20 servings Fresh Fruit

Dairy

◆ 3 Tbsp. Egg Substitute
◆ 1 cup 2 % Milk
◆ 4 tsp. Unsalted Butter
◆ 1 1/4 cup Non-fat Buttermilk
◆ Reduced-fat Cream Cheese
◆ Take Control Light Margarine
◆ 4 Eggs
◆ 1 oz. grated Parmigiano-Reggiano
3 oz. Low-fat Monterey Jack Cheese

Meat/Fish

2 – 4 ounce Halibut Filets
16 ounce Pork Tenderloin
4 – 4 ounces Boneless Skinless Chicken Breasts
8 ounces Sea Scallops
8 ounces Salmon Filet

Bakery

4 slices Sourdough Bread
1 Bagel

Pantry Items

Grand Marnier
◆ Splenda
◆ Pure Vanilla Extract
◆ Honey
◆ 1 Tbsp. Pine Nuts
◆ Salt
◆ Extra Virgin Olive Oil
◆ Black Pepper
1/4 cup White Wine
◆ Pure Maple Syrup
1 tsp. Curry Powder
10 threads Saffron
◆ Dark Sesame Oil
Seven Spice Seasoning
1/4 cup Lentils
◆ 1/4 cup Jasmine Rice
1 oz. Sun-dried Tomatoes
◆ 1 cup Non-fat Chicken Stock
◆ 1/2 cup Arborio Rice
◆ 1/8 tsp. Chili Powder
1 Tbsp. Dijon Mustard
10 oz. Plain Melba Toast
◆ 1 tsp. Dried Thyme
◆ 1 tsp. Dried Rosemary
◆ 1/2 tsp. Dried Oregano
◆ 1/4 tsp. Garlic Powder
◆ 1/2 tsp. Cayenne Pepper
1 small Dried Chipotle
Grapeseed Oil
1/4 tsp. Ground Cumin
1 Tbsp. Dijon Mustard
◆ 2 Tbsp. Capers
◆ 2 Tbsp. Balsamic Vinegar

Equipment

◆ Large Non-stick Skillet
◆ Muffin Pan
◆ Muffin Papers

◆ indicates previously purchased - check pantry first

Recipes

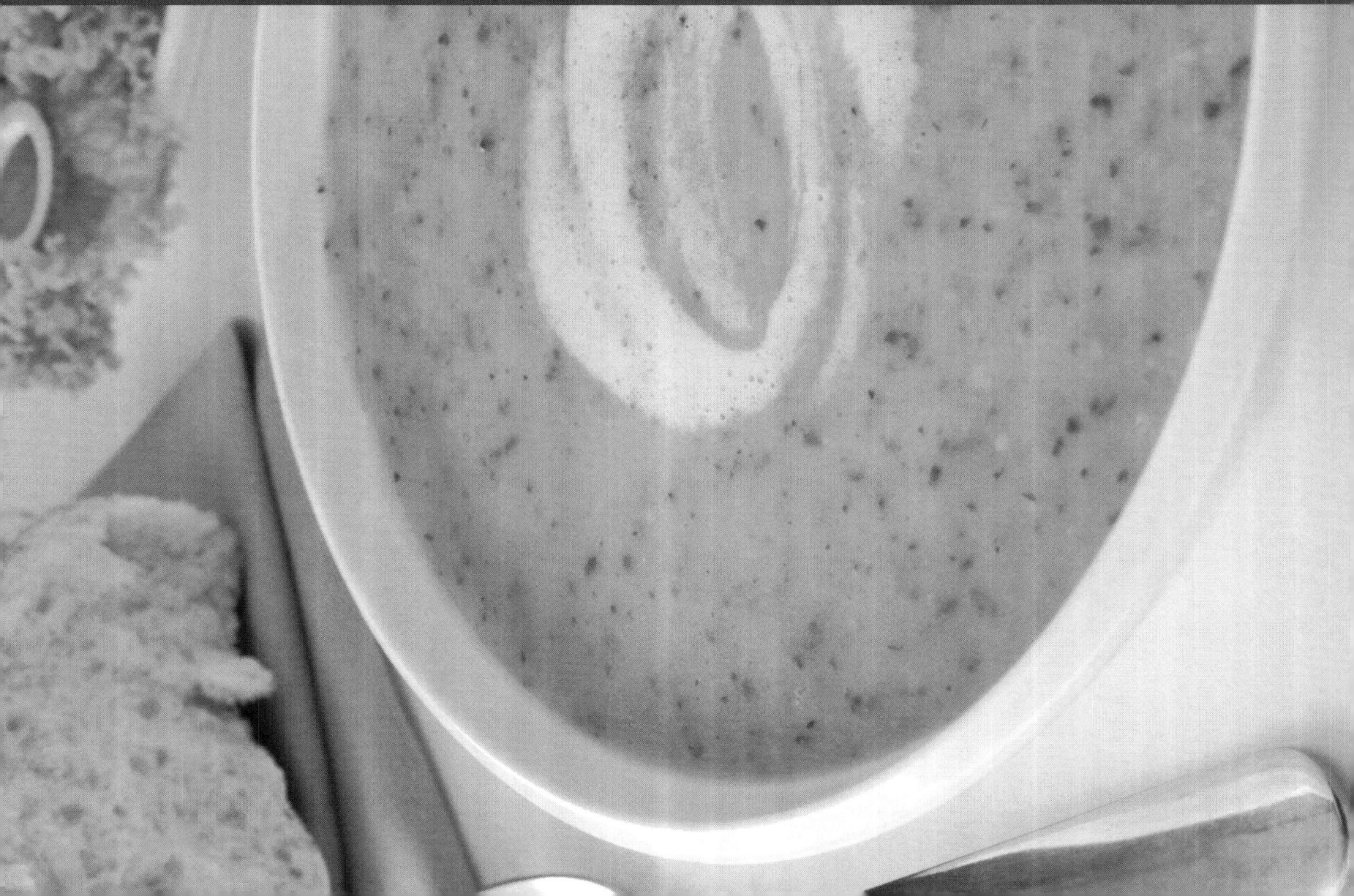

Apple Pancake

4 30 min.

Serving size = 1/4 pancake

I do not multiply this recipe but make two separate batches in two skillets. Leftovers are actually pretty good. Wrap tightly after cooled and refrigerate.

2 lbs. (4 medium)	granny smith apples
2 tsp.	unsalted butter
1/2 cup	Splenda
1/4 cup	water
3	large egg whites
1	large egg yolk
3/4 cup	non-fat buttermilk
3/4 cup	all purpose flour
1/4 tsp.	salt
2 Tbsp.	Splenda
2 tsp.	unsalted butter

Peel and core apples. Discard the peel. Slice very thin (about 1/8 inch thick).

Preheat oven to 425°F.

In a 12 inch iron skillet (or non-stick skillet) heat the butter, Splenda and water until boiling. Add apples and cook about 15 minutes. Stir the apples gently about every 3 minutes. As the apples cook the liquid will reduce and the mixture will turn a light golden brown caramel color. The bottom of the apples should be a caramel brown.

While the apples are cooking place the egg whites, egg yolk, buttermilk, flour, salt and the 2 tablespoons Splenda in a blender. Blend until smooth.

When the apples are caramelized pour the flour/buttermilk mixture over the apples so that the liquid covers them completely.

Transfer the pan to the oven and bake for about 15 – 18 minutes. The pancake is done when it is brown on top. It will puff slightly as it cooks.
Remove from the oven and place the 2 tsp. butter on top of the pancake to melt.

"If you want to make an apple pie from scratch, you must first create the universe..."
Carl Sagan

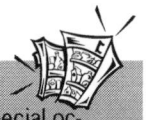

The refrigerator light goes on...
A dish like this one is perfect for a special occasion brunch. The best part is, if there are leftovers, they make good desserts a day or two later.

Nutrition Facts	
Serving size	1/4 pie
Servings	4
Calories 205	Calories from Fat 50
	% Daily Value
Total Fat 6 g	9 %
Saturated Fat 3 g	16 %
Trans Fat 0 g	
Monounsaturated Fat 2 g	
Cholesterol 64 mg	21 %
Sodium 237 mg	10 %
Total Carbohydrates 31 g	10 %
Dietary Fiber 2 g	10 %
Sugars 11 g	
Protein 8 g	
Vitamin A 4 %	Vitamin C 6 %
Calcium 7 %	Iron 7 %
Vitamin K 1 mcg	
Potassium 218 mg	
Magnesium 17 mg	

Blueberry Muffins

6 90 min.

Serving size = 1 muffin

This recipe can be multiplied by 2. Muffins will keep for 24 - 36 hours in a plastic bag. These freeze fairly well if sealed tightly in a plastic bag.

1	large egg
2 Tbsp.	reduced-fat spread
1/2 cup	Splenda
2 Tbsp .	non-fat yogurt
1/2 tsp.	pure vanilla extract
1 cup	all purpose flour
1/2 cup	whole wheat flour
2 Tbsp.	wheat germ
1/4 tsp.	salt
1 tsp.	baking powder
1/4 tsp.	baking soda
1/2 cup	non-fat buttermilk
1/2 cup	blueberries

Preheat oven to 375°F.

Separate the egg into an egg white and egg yolk. Set the egg yolk aside and whisk the egg white until frothy. Add the reduced-fat spread and whisk together until smooth. Add the Splenda®, egg yolk, yogurt and vanilla extract.

Whisk until smooth.

Place the all-purpose flour, whole wheat flour, wheat germ, salt, baking powder and baking soda in a sifter and sift into the mixing bowl.

Gently fold the creamed mixture together with the flour mixture. As this is blended, slowly add the buttermilk folding until smooth. As soon as the mixture is well blended, stop.

Gently fold the blueberries into the batter. Do not over mix.

Line a muffin tin with muffin papers and fill each muffin paper with an equal amount of batter. Bake for 12 – 15 minutes.

"Some people like cupcakes better. I, for one, care less for them!"

Frank Zappa, Musician

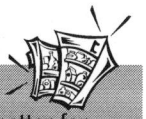

The refrigerator light goes on...
This is a great muffin that's so much better for you than a regular muffin. When I started with Dr. Gourmet I wanted to make food that people found familiar but healthier. This takes that a step further than the previous Blueberry Muffins posted on the web site because of the higher fiber content. One taster said that these "are so much better tasting than the original." That's what great food is – good food that just happens to be better for you.

Nutrition Facts	
Serving size	1 muffin
Servings	4
Calories 181	Calories from Fat 42
	% Daily Value
Total Fat 5 g	7 %
Saturated Fat 1 g	7 %
Trans Fat 0 g	
Monounsaturated Fat 2 g	
Cholesterol 36 mg	12 %
Sodium 296 mg	12 %
Total Carbohydrates 29 g	10 %
Dietary Fiber 2 g	10 %
Sugars 4 g	
Protein 6 g	
Vitamin A 5 %	Vitamin C 2 %
Calcium 9 %	Iron 10 %
Vitamin K 5 mcg	
Potassium 152 mg	
Magnesium 29 mg	

Scrambled Eggs

2 30 min.

Serving size = 2 eggs

This recipe can easily be multiplied by 2. Scrambled Eggs keep O.K. for about 24 hours and make great sandwiches with a bit of mayo, lettuce and tomato.

3	large egg whites
1	large egg yolk
2 Tbsp.	water
1/4 tsp.	salt
1 tsp.	unsalted butter
8 ounces	fresh crimini mushrooms (sliced)
	fresh ground black pepper

Place the egg whites, egg yolk, water and salt in a small mixing bowl and whisk until frothy.

Melt the butter in a small non-stick skillet pan over medium-high heat. Gently sauté the mushrooms until browned. Toss frequently. Cook the mushrooms until they are a dark caramel brown.

Add egg mixture and stir the eggs cooking until firm.

Add fresh ground black pepper to taste and serve.

"I myself prefer my New Zealand eggs for breakfast."
Elizabeth II, Queen of England 1952 - Present

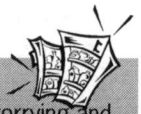

The refrigerator light goes on...
Eggs are good for you. Period. Quit worrying and enjoy them. You can substitute almost any veggie for the mushrooms but I like the meaty flavor that they bring. Scrambled eggs are especially good with red or green bell peppers.

Nutrition Facts	
Serving size	2 eggs
Servings	2
Calories 96	Calories from Fat 45
	% Daily Value
Total Fat 5 g	7 %
Saturated Fat 2 g	11 %
Trans Fat 0 g	
Monounsaturated Fat 2 g	
Cholesterol 110 mg	37 %
Sodium 383 mg	16 %
Total Carbohydrates 4 g	1 %
Dietary Fiber 1 g	4 %
Sugars 2 g	
Protein 10 g	
Vitamin A 4 %	Vitamin C 4 %
Calcium 2 %	Iron 5 %
Vitamin K 0 mcg	
Potassium 447 mg	
Magnesium 16 mg	

Blueberry Pancakes

2 30 min.

Serving size = 2 pancakes

This recipe can be halved or multiplied by 2 or 3. Leftover pancakes aren't very good. The batter will keep overnight but the pancakes will not be as good.

2/3 cup	all purpose flour
1 Tbsp.	Splenda
1 tsp	baking powder
2/3 cup	non-fat buttermilk
1/4 cup	egg substitute
1 tsp	pure vanilla extract
1/4 cup	fresh blueberries (or strawberries, blackberries)
2 tsp. (per serving)	Take Control Spread Light
1 Tbsp. (per serving)	pure maple syrup

Sift flour, Splenda and baking powder into a large mixing bowl.

Add buttermilk, egg substitute and vanilla extract and blend using a large whisk until smooth.

Heat a non-stick griddle over medium-high heat. Let the batter stand for at least 2 minutes while the griddle is heating. Stir once and wait another minute before placing batter on the griddle.

When the griddle is hot enough that a few drops of water will dance on the surface, reduce the heat to medium and place about 1/4 cup of batter for each pancake on the griddle.

After the pancakes have cooked for about a minute spread a tablespoon of fruit across the top of each one. Allow to cook for another 1 - 2 minutes until bubbles form on the surface and burst. Turn pancake and cook for about 1/2 the time of the first side until the are golden brown.

Remove and top with one teaspoon of Promise Buttery Spread Light on each pancake and serve one tablespoon of pure maple syrup for every two pancakes.

"Aspiring to a soufflé, he achieves a pancake at which the reader saws without much appetite."

John Leonard, Author

The refrigerator light goes on...

I love adding fruit to my pancakes. Any berry will do – blueberries, strawberries, blackberries – whatever is in the market. I have not had much success using frozen berries in my pancakes, however.

Nutrition Facts	
Serving size	2 pancakes (w/o fruit), with 2 tsp. Promise Buttery Spread Light and 1 Tbsp. pure maple syrup
Servings	2
Calories 294	Calories from Fat 49
	% Daily Value
Total Fat 6 g	9 %
Saturated Fat 1 g	7 %
Trans Fat 0 g	
Monounsaturated Fat 2 g	
Cholesterol 2 mg	1 %
Sodium 404 mg	17 %
Total Carbohydrates 50 g	17 %
Dietary Fiber 5 g	19 %
Sugars 14 g	
Protein 12 g	
Vitamin A 15 %	Vitamin C 4 %
Calcium 29 %	Iron 15 %
Vitamin K 7 mcg	
Potassium 468 mg	
Magnesium 75 mg	

Jean's French Toast

2 30 min.

Serving size = 2 slices bread

This recipe can easily be halved or doubled. Leftover French Toast is not very good. This batter doesn't keep well.

6 Tbsp.	egg substitute
2 tsp.	Splenda
6 Tbsp.	2% milk
1/4 tsp.	ground nutmeg
1/2 tsp.	pure vanilla extract
1/8 tsp.	salt
4 - 1 ounce slices	sourdough bread
2 tsp. (per serving)	Promise Buttery Spread Light
1 Tbsp.(per serving)	pure maple syrup

Place the egg substitute, Splenda, milk, ground nutmeg, vanilla and salt in a large mixing bowl. Whisk until well blended.

Heat a non-stick griddle over medium-high heat. When the griddle is hot enough that a few drops of water will dance on the surface, reduce the heat to medium and place 4 slices of bread into the batter. Gently dunk and turn the bread until it is well coated and slightly soaked.

Place the 4 slices of soaked bread on the griddle and cook for about 3 – 4 minutes. Turn and cook on the other side.

Cook, turning occasionally, until both sides are golden brown. Depending on your stove or griddle you may need to reduce the heat slightly.

Remove and top with one teaspoon of Promise Buttery Spread Light on each piece of toast and serve one tablespoon of pure maple syrup for every two slices of French toast.

"The menu said, 'Breakfast served any time'. So I ordered French Toast during the Renaissance."

Steven Wright, Comedian

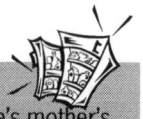

The refrigerator light goes on...

This French Toast is based on my wife's mother's recipe. She talked about it with such reverence that I was unsure about even cooking it. But I did.

I exchanged egg substitute for eggs and used 2% milk instead of whole milk. I also used Splenda instead of sugar. I didn't tell my wife of the changes and she didn't know when I served it to her.

The amazing thing about this recipe is the nutmeg. Most French Toast recipes use cinnamon, but the ground nutmeg creates a much more elegant flavor.

Nutrition Facts	
Serving size	2 slices French Toast w/2 tsp. Promise Buttery Spread Light and 1 Tbsp. pure maple syrup
Servings	2
Calories 346	Calories from Fat 65
	% Daily Value
Total Fat 7 g	11 %
Saturated Fat 2 g	161 %
Trans Fat 0 g	
Monounsaturated Fat 2 g	
Cholesterol 4 mg	1 %
Sodium 721 mg	30 %
Total Carbohydrates 55 g	18 %
Dietary Fiber 2 g	6 %
Sugars 19 g	
Protein 15 g	
Vitamin A 15 %	Vitamin C 0 %
Calcium 12 %	Iron 20 %
Vitamin K 4 mcg	
Potassium 355 mg	
Magnesium 31 mg	

Zucchini and Chévre Frittata

2 30 min.

Serving size = 1/2 pie

This recipe can be multiplied by 2 but requires a larger skillet. Leftovers are good. Wrap tightly after cooled and refrigerate. I like to make sandwiches from left over frittata.

1 medium	zucchini (sliced thin lengthwise)
	olive oil spray
1 tsp.	unsalted butter
1 clove	garlic (minced)
1/2	red onion (sliced)
2	large eggs
2	large egg whites
2 Tbsp.	water
1/8 tsp.	salt
2 Tbsp.	Parmigiano-Reggiano (grated)
1 ounce	semi soft goat cheese
	fresh ground black pepper

Preheat the oven to 425°F.

Place the zucchini on a non-stick cookie sheet and lightly spray with olive oil. Place the cookie sheet in the oven and roast the zucchini for about 7 – 10 minutes turning once. Remove and cool.

Heat 1/2 teaspoon butter in a small non-stick skillet over low-medium heat and add the garlic. Increase the heat and cook slowly over medium heat stirring frequently. Do not allow the garlic to brown. Add the sliced red onion and continue to cook until translucent. Set aside.

Whisk the eggs, egg whites, water and salt in a bowl until frothy. Fold in the Parmigiano-Reggiano.

Heat the remaining butter in a small non-stick skillet over high heat and when bubbling add the egg mixture. Reduce the heat to medium and simmer for about 2 minutes. Add the onion/garlic mixture distributing it across the top of the eggs.

Layer the zucchini slices on top in a crisscross pattern and then crumble the goat cheese over the top of the zucchini. Grind fresh pepper on top to taste.

Place in oven and cook for about 15 minutes until it puffs and is firm to the touch.

"Red onions are especially divine. I hold a slice up to the sunlight pouring in through the kitchen window, and it glows like a fine piece of antique glass. Cool watery-white with layers delicately edged with imperial purple...strong, humble, peaceful...with that fiery nub of spring green in the center..."

Mary Hayes Grieco

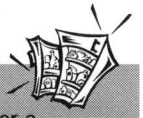

The refrigerator light goes on...
Just a little bit of rich cheese makes for a wonderfully rich recipe but doesn't add many calories.

Nutrition Facts	
Serving size	1/2 pie
Servings	2
Calories 211	Calories from Fat 113
	% Daily Value
Total Fat 13 g	20 %
Saturated Fat 7 g	33 %
Trans Fat 0 g	
Monounsaturated Fat 4 g	
Cholesterol 237 mg	79 %
Sodium 425 mg	18 %
Total Carbohydrates 9 g	3 %
Dietary Fiber 2 g	7 %
Sugars 4 g	
Protein 17 g	18 %
Vitamin A 15 %	Vitamin C 33 %
Calcium 15 %	Iron 9 %
Vitamin K 5 mcg	
Potassium 467 mg	
Magnesium 36 mg	

Blueberry Blue Cornmeal Pancakes

2 30 min.

Serving Size = 2 pancakes

This recipe can be halved or multiplied by 2 or 3. Leftover pancakes aren't very good. The batter will keep overnight but the pancakes will not be as good.

1/2 cup	blue cornmeal
1/4 cup	whole wheat flour
2 tsp.	Splenda
1 tsp.	baking powder
1/4 tsp.	salt
2/3 cups	non-fat buttermilk
1/4 cup	egg substitute
1 tsp.	pure vanilla extract
2 Tbsp. (per serving)	fresh blueberries
2 tsp. (per serving)	Take Control Light Spread
1 Tbsp. (per serving)	pure maple syrup

Place the blue cornmeal, whole wheat flour, Splenda, baking powder and salt in a sifter and sift into a medium sized mixing bowl. Add the buttermilk, egg substitute and vanilla extract and whisk until smooth.

Heat a non-stick griddle over medium-high heat. Let the batter stand for at least 2 minutes while the griddle is heating. Stir once and wait another minute before placing batter on the griddle.

When the griddle is hot enough that a few drops of water will sputter on the surface, reduce the heat to medium and place about 1/4 cup of batter for each pancake on the griddle.

After the pancakes have cooked for about a minute spread a tablespoon of blueberries across the top of each one. Allow to cook for another 1 - 2 minutes until bubbles form on the surface and burst. Turn pancake and cook for about 1/2 the time of the first side until they are golden brown.

Remove and top with one teaspoon of Take Control Light margarine on each pancake and serve one tablespoon of pure maple syrup for every two pancakes.

"Well, Art is Art, isn't it? Still, on the other hand, water is water. And east is east and west is west and if you take cranberries and stew them like applesauce they taste much more like prunes than rhubarb does. Now you tell me what you know."

Groucho Marx, Comedian

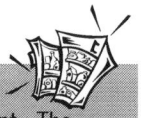

The refrigerator light goes on...
Never be afraid to use a new ingredient. The flavor of blue cornmeal is remarkably distinctive. It adds a new taste to a familiar comfort food.

Nutrition Facts

Serving size	2 pancakes w/2 tsp. Take Control Light Spread and 1 Tbsp. pure maple syrup
Servings	2
Calories 363	Calories from Fat 69
	% Daily Value
Total Fat 8 g	12 %
Saturated Fat 2 g	10 %
Trans Fat 0 g	
Monounsaturated Fat 2.5 g	
Cholesterol 4 mg	1 %
Sodium 322 mg	13 %
Total Carbohydrates 62 g	21 %
Dietary Fiber 6 g	23 %
Sugars 19 g	
Protein 13 g	
Vitamin A 12 %	Vitamin C 4 %
Calcium 20 %	Iron 16 %
Vitamin K 7 mcg	
Potassium 496 mg	
Magnesium 89 mg	

Four Grain Pancakes

2 30 min.

Serving size = 2 pancakes

This recipe can be halved or multiplied by 2 or 3. Leftover pancakes aren't very good. The batter will keep overnight but the pancakes will not be as good.

6 Tbsp.	whole wheat flour
6 Tbsp.	all purpose flour
3 Tbsp.	medium grind yellow corn meal
1/8 tsp.	salt
1 tsp.	baking powder
1 Tbsp.	Splenda
6 Tbsp.	old fashioned oatmeal
1 cup	non-fat buttermilk
1	large egg
2	large egg whites
2 tsp. (per serving)	Take Control Light Spread
1 Tbsp. (per serving)	pure maple syrup

Sift the whole wheat flour, all purpose flour, corn meal, salt and baking powder into a large mixing bowl.

Fold in the oatmeal.

Add the buttermilk and egg substitute and blend well until mixture is smooth.

Heat a non-stick griddle over medium-high heat. Let the batter stand for at least 2 minutes while the griddle is heating. Stir once and wait another minute before placing batter on the griddle.

When the griddle is hot enough that a few drops of water will dance on the surface, reduce the heat to medium and place about 1/4 cup of batter for each pancake on the griddle.

Cook until small bubbles on the surface of the pancake form and then burst. Turn and cook for about 1/2 the time that the pancakes cooked on the first side.

Remove and top with one teaspoon of Take Control Light Spread on each pancake and serve one tablespoon of pure maple syrup for every two pancakes.

"You have to eat oatmeal or you'll dry up. Anybody knows that."

Eloise, Star of Kay Thompson's Eloise books

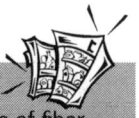

The refrigerator light goes on...
These are really good for you with tons of fiber, but because of the calories, best saved for a late Sunday brunch. You can also use flavored syrup.

Nutrition Facts

Serving size	2 pancakes (w/o fruit), w/2 tsp. Take Control Light Spread and 1 Tbsp. pure maple syrup
Servings	2
Calories 437	Calories from Fat 70
	% Daily Value
Total Fat 8 g	2 %
Saturated Fat 2 g	12 %
Trans Fat 0 g	
Monounsaturated Fat 3 g	
Cholesterol 107 mg	36 %
Sodium 469 mg	20 %
Total Carbohydrates 76 g	25 %
Dietary Fiber 6 g	24 %
Sugars 19 g	
Protein 17 g	
Vitamin A 18 %	Vitamin C 2 %
Calcium 34 %	Iron 20 %
Vitamin K 4 mcg	
Potassium 482 mg	
Magnesium 89 mg	

Tortilla

4 30 min.

Serving size = 1/4 pie

This recipe can be multiplied by 2 but requires a larger skillet. This recipe keeps well for about 24 – 48 hours and is good both cold and hot.

3 quarts	water
3/4 lb.	red potatoes
8	large egg whites
2	large egg yolks
1 Tbsp.	fresh curly or flat leaf parsley (minced)
1/4 tsp.	salt
2 tsp.	fresh oregano (minced)
1/8 tsp.	red pepper flakes
1/2 tsp.	jalapeño (minced)
	fresh ground black pepper to taste
2 tsp.	extra virgin olive oil
1	medium white onion (chopped)

Place the water in medium stock pot over high heat and bring to a boil. Reduce the heat to medium-high and cook the potatoes until slightly tender (about 20 minutes). Drain and let the potatoes cool slightly. Cut into 1/2 inch cubes.

Preheat the oven to 350°F.

Whisk together the egg whites, egg yolks, parsley, salt, oregano, red pepper flakes and minced jalapeño. Add fresh ground pepper to taste and then add the potatoes. Fold together gently until well blended.

Heat the olive oil in a 10 inch non-stick skillet over high heat and add the onions. Cook, stirring continuously, until soft and golden brown. Reduce the heat to medium and add the eggs/potato mixture.

Cook a two minutes on the stove and then transfer to the oven and cook for about twenty minutes (until the center is set).

"All happiness depends on a leisurely breakfast."
John Gunther

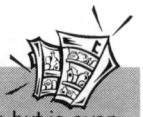

The refrigerator light goes on...
This dish is great right out of the oven but is even better the next day after it has chilled. This is the most common way that it is served in Spain and can be found all over the country in Tapas bars. Because the tortilla is made with eggs, be careful to keep it well chilled before serving.

Nutrition Facts	
Serving size	1/4 pie
Servings	4
Calories 153	Calories from Fat 43
	% Daily Value
Total Fat 5 g	7 %
Saturated Fat 1 g	6 %
Trans Fat 0 g	
Monounsaturated Fat 3 g	
Cholesterol 105 mg	35 %
Sodium 266 mg	11 %
Total Carbohydrates 17 g	6 %
Dietary Fiber 2 g	8 %
Sugars 3 g	
Protein 11 g	
Vitamin A 5 %	Vitamin C 18 %
Calcium 4 %	Iron 6 %
Vitamin K 21 mcg	
Potassium 551 mg	
Magnesium 30 mg	

Orange French Toast

2 30 min.

Serving size = 2 slices toast

This recipe can easily be doubled. Leftover French Toast is not very good. This batter doesn't keep well.

French Toast

3 Tbsp.	egg substitute
2 tsp.	Grand Marnier
1 tsp.	Splenda
1 Tbsp.	2% milk
1/4 tsp.	pure vanilla extract
1/4 cup	orange juice
1/4 tsp.	grated orange peel
4 slices	sourdough bread
2 tsp. (per serving)	Promise Buttery Spread Light

Orange Honey

2 Tbsp.	honey
1/2 tsp.	Grand Marnier

Place the egg substitute, Grand Marnier, Splenda, milk, vanilla extract, orange juice and orange peel in a medium-mixing bowl. Whisk until well blended.

Heat a non-stick griddle over medium-high heat. When the griddle is hot enough that a few drops of water will dance on the surface, reduce the heat to medium and place 4 slices of bread into the batter. Gently dunk and turn the bread until it is well coated and slightly soaked.

Place the 4 slices of soaked bread on the griddle and cook for about 3 – 4 minutes. Turn and cook on the other side.

Cook, turning occasionally, until both sides are golden brown. Depending on your stove or griddle you may need to reduce the heat slightly.

Remove and top with one teaspoon of Promise Buttery Spread Light on each piece of toast and serve one tablespoon of orange honey for every two slices of French toast.

"She was so wild that when she made French toast, she got her tongue caught in the toaster."

Rodney Dangerfield, Comedian

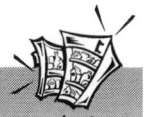

The refrigerator light goes on...
French Toast itself isn't all that bad for you. Just a few simple substitutions can make it even healthier by lowering the fat and cholesterol. Using 2% milk or the substitution of orange juice helps and the Take Control Light margarine reduces the calories dramatically. Enriched sauces, such as Orange Honey, can add different flavors to your pancakes or French toast.

Nutrition Facts

Serving size	2 slices French Toast w/2 tsp. Promise Buttery Spread Light and 1 Tbsp. orange honey
Servings	2
Calories 342	Calories from Fat 51
	% Daily Value
Total Fat 6 g	9 %
Saturated Fat 2 g	8 %
Trans Fat 0 g	
Monounsaturated Fat 2 g	
Cholesterol 1 mg	0 %
Sodium 523 mg	22 %
Total Carbohydrates 59 g	20 %
Dietary Fiber 2 g	7 %
Sugars 24 g	
Protein 11 g	
Vitamin A 13 %	Vitamin C 27 %
Calcium 5 %	Iron 17 %
Vitamin K 4 mcg	
Potassium 248 mg	
Magnesium 25 mg	

Orange Blueberry Scones

8 30 min.

Serving size = 1 scone

This recipe doesn't multiply well. The scones will keep sealed in plastic for about 36 hours. If refrigerated, they should also be sealed in plastic, and will keep for 96 hours.

2 cups	all purpose flour
1/4 cup	light brown sugar
2 tsp.	baking powder
1/2 tsp.	salt
2 Tbsp.	unsalted butter (softened)
1 tsp.	fresh grated orange peel
1/4 cup	orange juice
3/4 cup	non-fat buttermilk
1/4 cup	blueberries
2 Tbsp.	non-fat buttermilk
1 Tbsp.	light brown sugar

Preheat oven to 425°F.

Sift the flour, brown sugar, baking powder and salt into a large mixing bowl.

Cut in the softened butter with the tines of a fork or a pastry knife. It is well blended when the mixture is the consistency of coarse corn meal.

Add the orange juice and orange peel slowly while kneading the batter (I use a rubber spatula). Continue kneading while adding the buttermilk. The mixture will become a sticky dough.

Gently fold in the blueberries taking care not to let any burst.

Divide the dough into eight small triangles onto a non-stick cookie sheet.

Mix together the 2 Tbsp. buttermilk and 1 Tbsp. brown sugar and gently wash the tops of the scones. Place in the oven and bake for about 15 - 18 minutes until the tops of the scones are golden.

"When baking, follow directions. When cooking, go by your own taste."

Laiko Bahrs, Epicurean

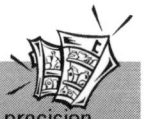

The refrigerator light goes on...
Ms. Bahrs is correct. Baking requires precision and care should be taken if making substitutions. This is because baking is essentially chemistry. There is more latitude with cooking, but when working with lower calorie recipes, sometimes even subtle changes can ruin a recipe.

Nutrition Facts	
Serving size	1 scone
Servings	8
Calories 188	Calories from Fat 30
	% Daily Value
Total Fat 3 g	5 %
Saturated Fat 2 g	10 %
Trans Fat 0 g	
Monounsaturated Fat 1 g	
Cholesterol 9 mg	3 %
Sodium 297 mg	12 %
Total Carbohydrates 35 g	12 %
Dietary Fiber 1 g	4 %
Sugars 10 g	
Protein 4 g	
Vitamin A 2 %	Vitamin C 5 %
Calcium 11 %	Iron 10 %
Vitamin K 1 mcg	
Potassium 123 mg	
Magnesium 14 mg	

Pumpkin Nut Muffins

6 30 min.

Serving size = 1 muffin

This recipe can be multiplied by 2. Muffins will keep for 24 hours in a plastic bag. To freeze muffins, wrap individually. Remove from bag for 20 minutes to thaw. Slice in half and reheat in an oven that has been preheated to 300°F.

1	large egg
2 Tbsp.	light spread (like Promise or Smart Balance)
1/2 cup	canned pumpkin
1/2 tsp.	pure vanilla extract
1/2 cup	Splenda
1/4 cup	dried pumpkin seeds
2 Tbsp.	golden seedless raisins
1 cup	all purpose flour
1/2 cup	whole wheat flour
2 Tbsp.	wheat germ
1/4 tsp.	salt
1 tsp.	baking powder
1/4 tsp.	baking soda
1/2 tsp.	ground nutmeg
1 tsp.	ground cinnamon
1/2 tsp.	ground allspice
1/3 cup	non-fat buttermilk
2 tsp.	light brown sugar

Preheat oven to 375°F.

Using a whisk, cream together the egg yolk and light spread. Add the pumpkin and whisk into the mixture until well blended. Add the vanilla extract and Splenda and blend. Fold in the pumpkin seeds and raisins.

Sift the all purpose flour, whole wheat flour, wheat germ, salt, baking powder, baking soda, nutmeg, cinnamon and allspice in a sifter and sift into the mixing bowl.

Gently fold the creamed mixture together with the flour mixture until smooth. When blended the mixture will still be dry. Whisk the egg white until it is white and foamy (about tripled in volume). Fold in the egg white.

Fold in the buttermilk and when the dough is just blended together stop.

Line a muffin tin with muffin papers and fill each muffin paper with an equal amount of batter. Place the muffins in the oven and bake for 20 minutes.

"It's the Great Pumpkin, Charlie Brown."
Linus

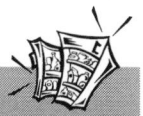

The refrigerator light goes on...
Make muffins on a weekend day for a grab and go healthy breakfast. These are simple to make, keep well for a few days and are not only delicious but have lots of fiber.

Nutrition Facts	
Serving size	1 muffin
Servings	12
Calories 206	Calories from Fat 52
	% Daily Value
Total Fat 6 g	9 %
Saturated Fat 1 g	7 %
Trans Fat 0 g	
Monounsaturated Fat 2 g	
Cholesterol 36 mg	12 %
Sodium 288 mg	12 %
Total Carbohydrates 32 g	11 %
Dietary Fiber 3 g	12 %
Sugars 5 g	
Protein 9 g	
Vitamin A 72 %	Vitamin C 2 %
Calcium 8 %	Iron 17 %
Vitamin K 8 mcg	
Potassium 237 mg	
Magnesium 64 mg	

Omelet

2 **30 min.**

Serving size = 1/2 omelet

This recipe is not easily multiplied. I do occasionally keep the other half of an omelet and make sandwiches with it.

1 tsp.	unsalted butter
1/3	bell pepper (julienne strips)
4	large egg whites
2	large egg yolks
1/8 tsp.	salt
3 Tbsp.	water
6	large fresh basil leaves
	fresh ground black pepper
1/2 ounce	Parmigiano-Reggiano (grated)

Melt the butter in a small non-stick skillet pan over medium heat. Add the peppers and cook until they are browned but not limp. Remove and set aside.

In a small mixing bowl whisk together the egg whites, eggs yolks, salt and water. Add ground pepper to taste.

Heat a medium sized non-stick skillet over medium-high heat and place the basil in the bottom and pour the egg mixture over the top. Reduce the heat to medium heat and cook slowly. Gently slide a spatula under the eggs and carefully fold back the cooked portion so as to expose more uncooked egg to the bottom of the pan.

When the eggs are nearly set, add the peppers to the center (in a straight line so as to make folding easier). Fold the omelet in half over the peppers. Cook about 2 more minutes and remove.

Sprinkle the Parmigiano-Reggiano over the top of the omelet and then divide into two portions.

"My wife and I tried to breakfast together, but we had to stop or our marriage would have been wrecked."

Winston Churchill, British Statesman

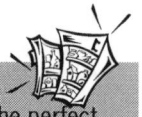

The refrigerator light goes on...
Don't read nutrition facts looking for the perfect 30% of calories from fat or so many grams of carbohydrates. It is what you eat in a day and not one particular dish that's important.

Nutrition Facts	
Serving size	1/2 omelet
Servings	2
Calories 144	Calories from Fat 77
	% Daily Value
Total Fat 9 g	13 %
Saturated Fat 4 g	20 %
Trans Fat 0 g	
Monounsaturated Fat 3 g	
Cholesterol 220 mg	73 %
Sodium 383 mg	16 %
Total Carbohydrates 3 g	1 %
Dietary Fiber 1 g	4 %
Sugars 1 g	
Protein 13 g	
Vitamin A 29 %	Vitamin C 27 %
Calcium 11 %	Iron 4 %
Vitamin K 9 mcg	
Potassium 260 mg	
Magnesium 29 mg	

Apple Cinnamon Bread

8 **45 min.**

Serving size = 1 slice

This recipe can be multiplied by 2. Bread will keep for 72 - 96 hours in a plastic bag. Reheat gently. This will freeze fairly well if sealed tightly in a plastic bag.

1/4 cup	pecans (coarsely chopped)
2 tsp.	maple syrup
1/4 tsp.	ground cinnamon
1	large egg yolk
1 Tbsp.	reduced-fat spread
2/3 cup	Splenda®
1/2 cup	unsweetened applesauce
1/2 tsp.	pure vanilla extract
3	large egg whites
1 1/4 cup	all purpose flour
3/4 cup	whole wheat flour
1/4 tsp.	salt
2 tsp.	baking powder
1/2 tsp.	baking soda
1 tsp.	ground cinnamon
1/4 cup	wheat germ
2 cups	apples (peeled and diced)
1/2 cup	non-fat buttermilk

Preheat oven to 350°F. Line a 1 1/2 quart glass Pyrex oblong loaf pan with foil (non-stick foil works best). Combine a the pecans, maple syrup and cinnamon in a small bowl. Stir until well blended. Set aside.

Whisk the egg yolk until smooth. Add the reduced- fat spread and whisk together until smooth. Add the Splenda, applesauce and vanilla extract and whisk until smooth.

In separate bowl whisk the egg whites until they begin to be very frothy and white. Do not beat into stiff peaks.

Place the all-purpose flour, whole wheat flour, salt, baking powder, baking soda, cinnamon and wheat germ in a sifter and sift into the mixing bowl.

Gently fold the creamed mixture together with the flour mixture. As this is blended add the grated apples. Just as the apples is blended in add buttermilk and fold until smooth. As soon as the mixture is well blended add the frothed egg whites and fold together until smooth. Pour the batter into the lined Pyrex dish and sprinkle the pumpkin seed mixture evenly over the top. Place the loaf pan in the preheated oven. Bake for 60 minutes.

"How many apples fell on Newton's head before he took the hint? Nature is always hinting at us. It hints over and over again. And suddenly we take the hint."

Robert Frost, Poet

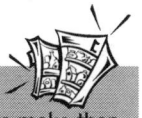

The refrigerator light goes on...
Making bread is a little more difficult to make than a simple muffin recipe. This Apple Cinnamon quick bread is a great comfort food. Warm and inviting with the spicy cinnamon aroma, just having this one in the oven makes the house more homey. The loaf will keep well for about 3 - 4 days and it's best to cut two thin slices and toast them lightly in the oven or toaster oven.

Nutrition Facts	
Serving size	1 slice
Servings	8
Calories 193	Calories from Fat 39
	% Daily Value
Total Fat 5 g	7 %
Saturated Fat 1 g	4 %
Trans Fat 0 g	
Monounsaturated Fat 2 g	
Cholesterol 27 mg	9 %
Sodium 312 mg	13 %
Total Carbohydrates 33 g	11 %
Dietary Fiber 3 g	13 %
Sugars 5 g	
Protein 7 g	
Vitamin A 3 %	Vitamin C 7 %
Calcium 9 %	Iron 11 %
Vitamin K 1 mcg	
Potassium 187 mg	
Magnesium 37 mg	

Curried Chicken Salad

3 30 min.

3 as a dinner entrée, 6 for lunch
Serving size = about 3/4 cup

This recipe can be multiplied by 2. This recipe keeps well for about 24 - 36 hours only. Serve with one 6 inch whole wheat pita round and garnish with cucumbers or alfalfa sprouts.

4 cups	water
4 ounce	boneless, skinless chicken breasts
1 tsp.	curry powder
2 Tbsp.	reduced-fat mayonnaise
1 Tbsp.	slivered almonds
2 Tbsp.	non-fat sour cream
1/8 tsp.	cinnamon
1 Tbsp.	chutney
2 Tbsp.	golden raisins
2 Tbsp.	green onions (chopped)
1/4 cup	celery (diced)
1 Tbsp.	red bell pepper (diced)

Place water in a shallow pan over high heat. When the liquid is at a shiver, reduce the heat to medium so that it won't boil. Add the chicken breasts and poach until just done. This should take about 10 minutes; check for an internal temperature of 170° to ensure the chicken is cooked.

When the chicken is cooked, remove it to a cutting board and let it cool for about 15 minutes; then put it in the refrigerator to chill.

When chilled, cube the chicken breasts and place in a medium mixing bowl. Add all the other ingredients and fold together until well coated.

Chill for at least an hour before serving.

"Chutney is marvelous. I'm mad about it. To me, it's very imperial."

Diana Vreeland, Editor
Vogue Magazine

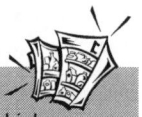

The refrigerator light goes on...
There are hundreds of ways to make chicken salad (or shrimp or tuna or etc.). Don't be timid. Mixing strong flavors, such as chutney, curry and raisins, makes for a rich taste while using less fat and calories.

Nutrition Facts	
Serving size	3/4 cup
Servings	3
Calories 141	Calories from Fat 46
	% Daily Value
Total Fat 5 g	8 %
Saturated Fat 1 g	4 %
Trans Fat 0 g	
Monounsaturated Fat 1 g	
Cholesterol 26 mg	9 %
Sodium 122 mg	5 %
Total Carbohydrates 14 g	5 %
Dietary Fiber 1 g	4 %
Sugars 9 g	
Protein 10 g	
Vitamin A 6 %	Vitamin C 11 %
Calcium 4 %	Iron 5 %
Vitamin K 27 mcg	
Potassium 244 mg	
Magnesium 23 mg	

Lentil and Black Bean Salad

3 45 min.

Serving size = about 1 1/2 cups

This recipe can easily be multiplied by 2. This salad keeps well for 3 – 4 days and is better the second day.

1/2 cup	red lentils
1/2 cup	green lentils
6 cups	water
1 – 15 ounce can	black beans (drained and rinsed)
1 large	shallot (minced)
1 rib	celery (sliced thin)
1/4 tsp.	red pepper flakes
1 Tbsp.	extra virgin olive oil
2 Tbsp.	white wine vinegar
1 Tbsp.	maple syrup
1 Tbsp.	curly parsley (chopped)
1/4 tsp.	salt
	ground black pepper to taste

Cook the red lentils in 3 cups of simmering water for about 15 – 20 minutes, until just tender. Drain and rinse with cold water.

Cook the green lentils in 3 cups of simmering water for about 15 – 20 minutes, until just tender. Drain and rinse with cold water.

Combine the green and red lentils with the black beans.

Add the shallot, celery, red bell pepper, olive oil, vinegar, maple syrup, parsley, salt and pepper.

Chill overnight.

"A man may be a pessimistic determinist before lunch and an optimistic believer in the will's freedom after it."

Aldous Huxley, Author

The refrigerator light goes on...
Lentils are amazingly high in fiber and taste great.

Nutrition Facts	
Serving size	1 1/2 cup
Servings	3
Calories 514	Calories from Fat 54
	% Daily Value
Total Fat 6 g	10 %
Saturated Fat 1 g	5 %
Trans Fat 0 g	
Monounsaturated Fat 4 g	
Cholesterol 0 mg	0 %
Sodium 220 mg	9 %
Total Carbohydrates 85 g	28 %
Dietary Fiber 30 g	119 %
Sugars 7 g	
Protein 31 g	
Vitamin A 7 %	Vitamin C 10 %
Calcium 3 %	Iron 47 %
Vitamin K 37 mcg	
Potassium 1677 mg	
Magnesium 195 mg	

Thai Cucumber Salad

Servings = 4
Serving size = about 1 cup salad as a side dish

This recipe can easily be multiplied by 2 or 3. Leftovers are good for 24 hours at the most.

1 cup	rice vinegar
1 tsp	lime zest
1/4 tsp.	Tabasco sauce
2 Tbsp.	Splenda
1/2 cup	red onion (diced)
2 large	cucumbers (peeled and sliced thin)
1/4 cup	cilantro leaves
1 Tbsp.	raw peanuts (chopped)

Combine the rice vinegar, lime zest, Tabasco, Spleda, red onion, cucumber slices and cilantro leaves in a glass or stainless steel bowl.

You can add the peanuts now and let them marinate. They will be slightly chewy, but I prefer to sprinkle them over the top of the salad when I am serving.

Marinate at least 2 hours.

"A spoonful of honey will catch more flies than a gallon of vinegar."

Benjamin Franklin,
American statesman

The refrigerator light goes on...
When I was a kid in Atlanta my mom used to make cucumbers and onions with white vinegar, a touch of salt and pepper and just enough sugar to take the bite off. The flavors are the same – Southeast America, Southeast Asia – just subtle differences.

Nutrition Facts	
Serving size	1 cup salad
Servings	4
Calories 46	Calories from Fat 11
	% Daily Value
Total Fat 1 g	2 %
Saturated Fat <1 g	1 %
Trans Fat 0 g	
Monounsaturated Fat 0 g	
Cholesterol 0 mg	0 %
Sodium 8 mg	0 %
Total Carbohydrates 5 g	2 %
Dietary Fiber 1 g	5 %
Sugars 3 g	
Protein 1 g	
Vitamin A 3 %	Vitamin C 10 %
Calcium 3 %	Iron 3 %
Vitamin K 10 mcg	
Potassium 229 mg	
Magnesium 21 mg	

Mediterranean Chicken Salad

4 45 min.

Serving size = about 2 cups salad

This recipe can easily be multiplied by 2. It makes great leftovers and is actually better the second day. Keep in refrigerator for no more than 48 hours.

1 clove	garlic minced
1 lb.	boneless chicken breasts (sliced into thin strips)
	spray olive oil
1 large	red onion (sliced)
1/2	red bell pepper (sliced into thin strips)
1/2	yellow bell pepper (sliced into thin strips)
1 small	zucchini (cut into large dice)
8 oz.	grape tomatoes
1 Tbsp.	extra virgin olive oil & honey
2 Tbsp.	balsamic vinegar
1/2 tsp.	salt
to taste	fresh ground black pepper
12	black olives (cut in quarters)
8 leaves	fresh basil (chiffonade)
8 leaves	romaine lettuce
1 - 2 oz. (per serving)	whole wheat roll
1/2 oz. (per serving)	goat cheese

Preheat oven to 350°F. Place a large non-stick grill pan and a large non-stick skillet in the oven. (Two large non-stick skillets will do.).

While the oven is heating combine the minced garlic and chicken breast strips in a bowl and place the bowl in the refrigerator.

When the pans are hot spray each lightly with olive oil and add the sliced red onion to the grill pan and the zucchini and grape tomatoes to the skillet. Cook the tomatoes and zucchini for about 5 to 7 minutes tossing twice to make sure that they are well seared. Remove before the tomatoes get soft and place in a large bowl to cool in the refrigerator. Return the skillet to the oven.

Cook the onions tossing frequently until they begin to brown. Add the red and yellow pepper strips and cook for about 5 to 7 minutes tossing once or twice. Remove before the peppers get too soft and add to the cooling tomato/zucchini mixture and toss well.

Spray the large skillet lightly again with olive oil and add the garlic and chicken strips. Cook for about 10 minutes tossing once or twice. Make sure the chicken is cooked through. Remove and add to the roasted vegetable mixture tossing to coat well.
Add the olive oil, balsamic vinegar, honey, salt, pepper, olives and basil. Toss to coat the salad well and then return to the refrigerator to chill for at least 2 hours. When ready to serve cut the romaine lettuce into strips and fold into the salad.

Slice the rolls and then heat gently. Serve spread with goat cheese.

"The whole Mediterranean ... the wine, the ideas ... seems to ride in the sour pungent taste of those black olives ... A taste older than meat, older than wine. A taste as old as cold water."

Lawrence Durrell, Author, Playwright

Nutrition Facts	
Serving size	2 cups w/rolls and goat cheese
Servings	4
Calories 422	Calories from Fat 109
	% Daily Value
Total Fat 12 g	4 %
Saturated Fat 4 g	1 %
Trans Fat 0 g	
Monounsaturated Fat 0 g	
Cholesterol 0 mg	0 %
Sodium 149 mg	6 %
Total Carbohydrates 9 g	3 %
Dietary Fiber 4 g	16 %
Sugars 3 g	
Protein 1 g	
Vitamin A 1 %	Vitamin C 33 %
Calcium 1 %	Iron 3 %
Vitamin K 2 mcg	
Potassium 143 mg	
Magnesium 12 mg	

Jicama Salad

Servings = 8
Serving size = 1 cup salad
This recipe can easily be halved or multiplied by 2.
Keeps well for 2 – 3 days in the refrigerator.

1 medium	jicama root (matchstick)
2	limes (juiced)
1/2 tsp.	salt
2 tsp.	maple syrup
1/4 cup	cilantro leaves
1/2 tsp.	ground cumin
4 tsp.	grapeseed oil

After peeling and cutting the jicama into matchstick place it in a large glass or stainless steel bowl with the lime juice, salt, maple syrup, cilantro, cumin and grapeseed oil. Toss well and chill for at least 2 hours before serving.

"The best way to lose weight is to close your mouth - something very difficult for a politician. Or watch your food - just watch it, don't eat it."

Edward Koch, former
mayor of New York City

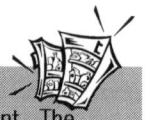

The refrigerator light goes on...
Never be afraid to use a new ingredient. The crunch of jicama makes great salads. Its sweet flavor goes great in salads when used raw but works well in soups and stews much like a turnip or parsnip.

Nutrition Facts	
Serving size	1 cup salad
Servings	8
Calories 59	Calories from Fat 21
	% Daily Value
Total Fat 2 g	4 %
Saturated Fat 0 g	1 %
Trans Fat 0 g	
Monounsaturated Fat 0 g	
Cholesterol 0 mg	0 %
Sodium 149 mg	6 %
Total Carbohydrates 9 g	3 %
Dietary Fiber 4 g	16 %
Sugars 3 g	
Protein 1 g	
Vitamin A 1 %	Vitamin C 33 %
Calcium 1 %	Iron 3 %
Vitamin K 2 mcg	
Potassium 143 mg	
Magnesium 12 mg	

Spaghetti Squash Salad

Servings = 8
Serving size = about one cup.

This recipe can easily be halved. 90 minutes total time and 30 minutes actual cooking time. This recipe keeps well for up to 3 days.

2 quarts	water
1	spaghetti squash
3 Tbsp.	olive oil
4 tsp.	balsamic vinegar
1 Tbsp.	pure maple syrup
1 medium	red bell pepper (diced)
1 large	shallot (minced)
1/2 tsp.	salt
to taste	fresh ground black pepper

Place the water in a large stock pot over high heat.

When the water is boiling add the spaghetti squash and reduce the heat to a slow boil. Cook for 25 minutes and remove from the water. Let the squash rest on the counter to cool.

Cut the cooled squash open lengthwise and remove the seeds. Scoop out the flesh of the squash gently dividing the strands.

Toss the squash with the olive oil, vinegar, maple syrup, red pepper, shallot, salt and pepper. Chill well.

"Prince Charles is very relaxed at the table, throwing his salad around willy-nilly. I didn't find him stiff at all."

Madonna, Singer

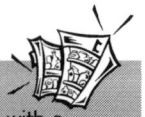

The refrigerator light goes on...
This is a perfect lunch salad. Pair this with a hearty whole grain roll lightly toasted and smeared with just a bit of cheese and you can taste the summer any time of year.

Nutrition Facts	
Serving size	1 cup
Servings	4
Calories 118	Calories from Fat 51
	% Daily Value
Total Fat 6 g	9 %
Saturated Fat 1 g	4 %
Trans Fat 0 g	
Monounsaturated Fat 4 g	
Cholesterol 0 mg	0 %
Sodium 164 mg	7 %
Total Carbohydrates 17 g	6 %
Dietary Fiber 1 g	4 %
Sugars 5 g	
Protein 2 g	
Vitamin A 32 %	Vitamin C 96 %
Calcium 4 %	Iron 5 %
Vitamin K 5 mcg	
Potassium 289 mg	
Magnesium 24 mg	

Roasted Eggplant Salad

Servings = 8
Serving size = about one cup.

This recipe can easily be multiplied by 2. or halved. This recipe keeps well in the refrigerator for about 72 hours.

	spray olive oil
2 lbs.	eggplant (cut into 1/2 inch cubes)
2 medium	yellow onions (cut into 1/8th wedges)
1 pint	grape tomatoes
1/4 cup	slivered almonds
1/2 tsp.	salt
to taste	fresh ground black pepper
2 Tbsp.	extra virgin olive oil
3 Tbsp.	balsamic vinegar
1/4 cup	fresh basil (chiffonade)
1 Tbsp.	fresh oregano
1 bulb	roasted garlic (chopped)

Preheat oven to 325°F. Place a large roasting pan in the oven. When the oven is hot lightly spray the pan with oil and add the eggplant, onions, tomatoes and almonds.

Return the pan to the oven and roast for about 30 - 40 minutes. Stir the vegetables about every 10 minutes. They may require a light spray once or twice with the oil to keep them from sticking.

Remove form the oven and let the vegetables cool slightly. Place in a large mixing bowl and add the salt, pepper, olive oil, vinegar, basil, oregano and roasted garlic.

Stir well and chill.

** The garlic can be roasted at the same time as the vegetables using the Roasted Garlic recipe. Alternatively, add 5 cloves of minced garlic with the veggies before roasting. The flavor will be less subtle but is quite good (and the recipe is easier if you haven't roasted the garlic).

"How can people say they don't eat eggplant when God loves the color and the French love the name? I don't understand."

Jeff Smith, The Frugal Gourmet

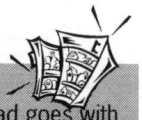

The refrigerator light goes on...
This is a very easy recipe and the salad goes with everything. You can serve it under fish or with a pasta recipe as a side dish. It's great to take to a pot luck and everyone will love you for it (and they don't even have to know that it's healthy).

Nutrition Facts	
Serving size	1 cup
Servings	4
Calories 118	Calories from Fat 58
	% Daily Value
Total Fat 7 g	10 %
Saturated Fat 1 g	4 %
Trans Fat 0 g	
Monounsaturated Fat 4 g	
Cholesterol 0 mg	0 %
Sodium 151 mg	6 %
Total Carbohydrates 14 g	5 %
Dietary Fiber 5 g	22 %
Sugars 5 g	
Protein 3 g	
Vitamin A 7 %	Vitamin C 16 %
Calcium 5 %	Iron 5 %
Vitamin K 14 mcg	
Potassium 445 mg	
Magnesium 41 mg	

Black Eyed Pea Salad

Servings = 4
Serving size = about one cup.

This recipe can easily be multiplied by 2 or 3. This recipe is better if made the night before and it keeps well for about 48 hours in the fridge.

3 quarts	water
2 1/3 cups	dried black eyed peas
1 medium	carrot (peeled and diced)
1 rib	celery (diced)
2 Tbsp.	red onion (minced)
1/3	green bell pepper (seeded and diced)
1 Tbsp.	grapeseed oil
1 Tbsp.	pure maple syrup
2 Tbsp.	apple cider vinegar
1/2 tsp.	salt
1/8 tsp.	fresh ground black pepper
2 Tbsp.	fresh dill (chopped)

Rinse the peas well and place in a large pot. Cover with cold water and soak overnight if possible. Drain the peas and replace with 3 quarts of cold water. Cook the peas for about an hour.

** An alternative quick method is to place the peas in a pot and cover with cold water. Bring to a boil and cook for two minutes. Remove the peas from the heat rinse and lest stand one hour. Rinse and place in a pot with 3 quarts of cold water. Cook the peas for about an hour until soft.

** Canned no salt added black eyed peas may be used. Rinse well. You will need two 15 ounce cans for this recipe.

When the beans are cooked, drain well and cool. Place in a medium mixing bowl and add the carrot, celery, bell pepper, grapeseed oil, maple syrup, vinegar, salt, pepper and fresh dill. Toss well and chill at least an hour.

"The South is the only place in the world where nothing has to be explained to me."

Woodrow Wilson, 28th
President of the USA

The refrigerator light goes on...
You wouldn't think that black eyed peas are all that good for you but they are. The cheap, lowly black eye is a member of the legume family and chock full of everything good for you. A great ingredient as a side dish with your Oven Fried Chicken or used in a salad.

Nutrition Facts	
Serving size	1 cup
Servings	4
Calories 208	Calories from Fat 36
	% Daily Value
Total Fat 4 g	6 %
Saturated Fat 1 g	3 %
Trans Fat 0 g	
Monounsaturated Fat 1 g	
Cholesterol 0 mg	0 %
Sodium 320 mg	13 %
Total Carbohydrates 33 g	11 %
Dietary Fiber 9 g	38 %
Sugars 9 g	
Protein 10 g	
Vitamin A 55 %	Vitamin C 24 %
Calcium 5 %	Iron 19 %
Vitamin K 10 mcg	
Potassium 499 mg	
Magnesium 75 mg	

Pizza with Tomato, Basil and Roasted Garlic

3 **30 min.**

Serving size = 1 individual pizza

This recipe can easily be multiplied by 2, 3 or 4. Leftovers are good cold for breakfast. This recipe requires Whole Wheat Pizza Dough and Roasted Garlic to be made first (recipes included).

1 medium (4 ounce)	tomato
1 ounce	fresh mozzarella
8 large	fresh basil leaves
4 cloves	roasted garlic
1/2 ounce	Parmigiano-Reggiano (grated)
1/4	whole wheat pizza dough

Preheat the oven to 500°F.

Pizza is best baked on a pizza stone but a cookie sheet will work as well. Place the baking stone or cookie sheet in the oven and allow it to heat at least 15 - 20 minutes.

While the baking surface is heating, slice tomato in half vertically. Remove the seeds and slice the tomato into julienne strips.

Cut the fresh mozzarella into 1/2 inch cubes.

Gently slice the basil into strips.

Cut each clove of roasted garlic into quarters.

Gently toss the tomato strips, mozzarella, basil leaves and garlic together in a small mixing bowl.

Set the tomato mixture close to the oven so that it will be accessible and easy to place on top of the dough. Have the grated parmesan within easy reach.

Using 1/4 of the pizza dough recipe (for each pizza) gently stretch into 8-inch rounds. Don't work too hard to get a perfectly round shape.

Once the dough is formed, place it on the hot pizza stone and top with the tomato/mozzarella mixture.

Bake for approximately eight minutes, and then top with the Parmesan cheese. Bake for another 3 – 5 minutes - until the cheese has melted. Remove from the oven and let it cool for about 90 seconds, slice and serve.

"Never eat more than you can lift."
Miss Piggy

The refrigerator light goes on...
A pizza stone is the key to baking a professional quality pie. They are inexpensive and so worth using.

Nutrition Facts	
Serving size	1 pizza (includes dough and toppings)
Servings	1
Calories 479	Calories from Fat 109
	% Daily Value
Total Fat 12 g	19 %
Saturated Fat 6 g	32 %
Trans Fat 0 g	
Monounsaturated Fat 4 g	
Cholesterol 32 mg	11 %
Sodium 708 mg	30 %
Total Carbohydrates 73 g	24 %
Dietary Fiber 10 g	40 %
Sugars 11 g	
Protein 24 g	
Vitamin A 13 %	Vitamin C 35 %
Calcium 41 %	Iron 31 %
Vitamin K 24 mcg	
Potassium 713 mg	
Magnesium 125 mg	

Whole Wheat Pizza Dough

Servings = enough dough for 4 individual pizzas
Serving size = 1 individual pizza

This recipe is easily multiplied by 2 or cut in half. This dough will keep for about 36 hours in the refrigerator if wrapped tightly in plastic wrap. It will not be as good as fresh.

1 cup	warm water
1 tsp.	dry active yeast
4 tsp.	honey
2 cups	whole wheat flour (does not need to be sifted)
1/2 cup	all purpose flour (does not need to be sifted)
1/2 tsp.	salt

Heat the water in the microwave until warm to touch – about 110°F to 115°F. (I prefer to use a thermometer for this because if the water is too hot you will kill the yeast.)

Place the yeast and honey in a large mixing bowl and pour the heated water over the mixture, stirring until well blended. Let the mixture stand for about 5 - 7 minutes until foamy.

Add the whole wheat flour, all purpose flour and salt and stir with a fork until a coarse dough forms.

Continue to mix by hand until a dough ball forms and all the flour is well blended.

Cover the bowl and place it in a sink with about 4 inches of hot water in the bottom.The heat from the warm water will help the dough rise. The dough will double in size in about 30 – 40 minutes. Punch it a few times with your fingers and let it rise another 30 minutes.

Remove from the bowl and cut the ball into four equal pieces. Cover the dough that you are not going to use immediately in plastic wrap and chill.

"Blues is to jazz what yeast is to bread. Without it, it's flat."

Carmen McRae, Singer

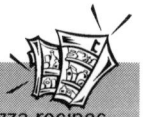

The refrigerator light goes on...
Using whole wheat pizza dough for pizza recipes is a great way to get extra fiber. The dough has more body than regular pizza dough and a mellow, sweet flavor. And it adds 6 grams of fiber to your diet!

Nutrition Facts	
Serving size	1 pizza
Servings	4
Calories 284	Calories from Fat 9
	% Daily Value
Total Fat 1 g	5 %
Saturated Fat 0 g	0 %
Trans Fat 0 g	
Monounsaturated Fat 0 g	
Cholesterol 0 mg	0 %
Sodium 295 mg	12 %
Total Carbohydrates 61 g	20 %
Dietary Fiber 8 g	32 %
Sugars 6 g	
Protein 10 g	
Vitamin A 0 %	Vitamin C 0 %
Calcium 2 %	Iron 18 %
Vitamin K 1 mcg	
Potassium 283 mg	
Magnesium 87 mg	

Roasted Garlic

Servings = 6
Serving Size = 1/3 head of garlic (about 6 cloves)

I make up to about 4 heads of garlic at a time. This keeps well, tightly covered, for about 4 – 6 days.

2 heads	whole garlic
2 tsp.	extra virgin olive oil

Preheat oven to 300°F.

Peel the outermost skin of the garlic only. With the bulb whole, turn on its side and slice 1/2-inch of the stem end off the garlic bulbs.

Pour the olive oil in the bottom of a heavy bottom sauce pan.

Place the garlic cut side down in the pan.

Cover and roast for 45 minutes until cloves are slightly brown at the cut end and soft throughout.

There is no such thing as a little garlic.
Arthur Baer, Investment Author

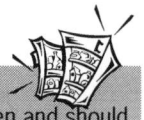

The refrigerator light goes on...
Roasted garlic is a staple in my kitchen and should be in yours. I generally roast about 3 heads every ten days or so. It makes a great ingredient in mashed potatoes and also enriches any sauce. It is fantastic served as hors d'oeuvres on bread with some soft goat cheese and veggies.

Nutrition Facts	
Serving size	1/3 head of garlic (about 4 cloves)
Servings	6
Calories 40	Calories from Fat 14
	% Daily Value
Total Fat 2 g	2 %
Saturated Fat 0 g	1 %
Trans Fat 0 g	
Monounsaturated Fat 0 g	
Cholesterol 0 mg	0 %
Sodium 3 mg	0 %
Total Carbohydrates 6 g	2 %
Dietary Fiber 0 g	2 %
Sugars 0 g	
Protein 1 g	
Vitamin A 0 %	Vitamin C 9 %
Calcium 3 %	Iron 2 %
Vitamin K 1 mcg	
Potassium 72 mg	
Magnesium 5 mg	

Butternut Squash Risotto

4 **45 min.**

Serving size = about 2 cups

This recipe can easily be multiplied by 2. Leftovers are good. Reheat gently.

2 lbs	butternut squash
	spray olive oil
2 tsp	extra virgin olive oil
1 large	leek
1/2 medium	red onion (diced)
1 cup	arborio rice
3 cups	water
1 cup	low sodium chicken or vegetable broth
1/4 cup	dry sherry
1/4 tsp	salt
to taste	fresh ground black pepper
1/4 tsp	ground paprika
1 1/2 ounces	Parmigiano-Reggiano (grated)
1 Tbsp	Italian parsley leaves

Preheat the oven to 325°F.

Slice the squash lengthwise and remove the seeds. Spray lightly with olive oil and place in the preheated oven, cut side up. Roast the squash for about 1 hour, until slightly tender.

Remove from the oven and let cool. The squash will have a small amount of liquid in the cavity. After it is cool, drain the liquid and place the squash on a cutting board, cut side down.

Gently peel the skin away from the squash. Slice across the squash parallel to the cutting board, dividing into three slices. Keep the shape of the squash intact. Slice lengthwise at about 1/4 inch intervals and then crosswise, so as to divide into 1/2 inch cubes. Set aside.

Slice the root off of the leek. Slice the leek in half, separating the white from the green tops. Clean the green tops under running water and slice very thin. Slice the white part of the leek very thin lengthwise and clean well.

Heat the olive oil in a large sauce pan over high heat and add the green part of the leek. Reduce the heat to medium-high and cook very slowly. Stir frequently.

When the leek is wilted, add the white part of the leek and the diced red onion. Reduce the heat to medium and cook for about five minutes, until the onions begin to soften.

Place the rice in the pan with the onions and leeks and stir for about 3 minutes. Add two cups of water, the chicken stock, sherry, salt and pepper. Cook over medium-high heat stirring frequently. Add the remaining water, 1 cup at a time.

Add the ground paprika and continue cooking. The rice will take about 20 to 25 minutes to cook and may require more water be added. Stir frequently, using about 1/2 cup of water at a time as needed, until the rice is soft but not mushy and there is a small amount of creamy sauce.

Stir in the Parmigiano-Reggiano until it is melted and then gently fold in the diced butternut squash and parsley.

Nutrition Facts	
Serving size	About 2 cups risotto
Servings	4
Calories 394	Calories from Fat 52
	% Daily Value
Total Fat 6 g	10 %
Saturated Fat 2 g	4 %
Trans Fat 0 g	
Monounsaturated Fat 3 g	
Cholesterol 7 mg	0 %
Sodium 348 mg	6 %
Total Carbohydrates 73 g	5 %
Dietary Fiber 7 g	22 %
Sugars 8 g	
Protein 11 g	
Vitamin A 487 %	Vitamin C 16 %
Calcium 25 %	Iron 5 %
Vitamin K 30 mcg	
Potassium 970 mg	
Magnesium 103 mg	

Seared Tuna Steak with Sake-Wasabi Sauce

2 **30 min.**

Serving size = 4 ounce tuna steak

This recipe can easily be multiplied by 2 but requires two large pans. Leftover tuna makes great tuna sandwiches or salads. Serve with Brown Rice (recipe included).

2 tsp.	low-sodium soy sauce
1 Tbsp.	sake
1 Tbsp.	freshly lime juice
2 Tbsp.	honey
1 tsp.	wasabi paste
2 - 4 ounce	tuna steaks (about 1 1/2 inch thick)
1/8 tsp.	salt
	fresh ground black pepper
1 tsp.	dark sesame oil

Mix the soy sauce, sake, lime juice, honey and wasabi paste together in a small bowl. Whisk until the wasabi is completely dissolved. This can be done a day in advance and refrigerated.

Rinse the tuna steaks and pat dry. Sprinkle one side with the salt and then pepper liberally on that side.

Place the sake sauce in a small sauce pan and heat over low heat. Do not allow the sauce to boil.

Set the oven to warm and place serving plates inside.

Heat the sesame oil in a large non-stick skillet over high until very hot (almost smoking). Add the tuna steaks, seasoned side down. Cook over medium-high heat until well seared and turn. Rare tuna will take about 4 - 5 minutes per side.

Remove the plates from the oven and spoon about 4 tablespoons of the heated sauce into the bottom of each plate.

This dish is made to be served with Brown Rice (recipe included) but any rice will do. When the tuna is done mound a serving of rice in the center of the plate on top of the sauce and place the tuna on top. Garnish by sprinkling the chopped scallions over the fish and serve.

"Catch a man a fish, and you can sell it to him. Teach a man to fish, and you ruin a wonderful business opportunity."

Karl Marx, well known communist

The refrigerator light goes on...
Searing any meat, such as tuna, makes for a rich and luxurious dish and is a healthy cooking technique. Make sure that the pan is very hot and add the meat carefully so as to not splash any hot oil.

Nutrition Facts	
Serving size	1 tuna steak
Servings	4
Calories 227	Calories from Fat 30
	% Daily Value
Total Fat 3 g	5 %
Saturated Fat 1 g	3 %
Trans Fat 0 g	
Monounsaturated Fat 1 g	
Cholesterol 51 mg	17 %
Sodium 372 mg	15 %
Total Carbohydrates 20 g	7 %
Dietary Fiber 1 g	3 %
Sugars 18 g	
Protein 27 g	
Vitamin A 4 %	Vitamin C 12 %
Calcium 4 %	Iron 7 %
Vitamin K 32 mcg	
Potassium 587 mg	
Magnesium 64 mg	

Linguine with Shrimp in Vodka Tomato Cream Sauce

4 **45 min.**

Serving Size = 2 ounces pasta/4 ounces shrimp

This recipe can easily be multiplied by 2 if you use a large skillet. Leftovers are fair at best. This recipe requires the Tomato Sauce (recipe inc luded) to be made first.

1 cup	water
1/2 cup	sun-dried tomatoes sliced
3 cups	water
16 spears	asparagus
4 tsp.	unsalted butter
1 lb.	large shrimp (peeled & deveined)
1 cup	shallots (sliced)
1/2 cup	vodka
1 cup	tomato sauce (recipe included)
1 cup	2% milk
1/4 tsp.	salt
5 quarts	water
8 ounces	linguine
2 Tblsp	fresh basil (chiffonade)

Heat 1 cup water until boiling and pour over the sun-dried tomatoes. Allow to stand for about 15 minutes, until soft and then drain the liquid into a sauce pan. Heat the liquid on high heat until it boils and reduce to 1/4 cup. Set aside.

Heat 3 cups of water to the shiver stage in a medium skillet. Add the asparagus and blanch for about 2 – 3 minutes, until they just begin to turn bright green. Remove and let dry on a paper towel. When they are cool, cut them in 2 inch segments.

Melt the butter in a large skillet over medium-high heat. Add the shrimp and sauté until slightly firm (no more than about 2 minutes on each side). Remove shrimp to a plate.

Begin heating the 5 quarts of water in a large pot. Add the linguine and cook about 15 minutes until just done (the pasta should have a slightly firm texture).

As the pasta is cooking, add the shallots to the skillet and cook over medium heat until they begin to soften and turn slightly brown (about 7 - 10 minutes).

Reduce the heat to low, add the vodka and cook briefly; then add the reduced water from the sun dried tomatoes, tomato sauce, milk and salt. After this has cooked for about 3 minutes, add the asparagus and sun-dried tomatoes. Simmer until tomatoes are tender (about 4 minutes). Add shrimp; toss to coat and allow to cook for another 4 minutes, until the shrimp is heated through.

Drain the linguine. Add the pasta to the tomato sauce and toss to coat well. Season to taste with fresh ground black pepper.

Served topped with basil.

The refrigerator light goes on...
519 calories may seem like a lot, but look carefully at the Nutrition Facts. This is a whole meal and it has so much going for it. It is low in fat and cholesterol, and has tomatoes, asparagus, tons of vitamins, and lycopenes– all in one pasta bowl.

Nutrition Facts	
Serving size	2 oz. pasta/4 oz. shrimp
Servings	4
Calories 519	Calories from Fat 72
	% Daily Value
Total Fat 8 g	13 %
Saturated Fat 4 g	19 %
Trans Fat 0 g	
Monounsaturated Fat 2 g	
Cholesterol 185 mg	62 %
Sodium 500 mg	21 %
Total Carbohydrates 60 g	22 %
Dietary Fiber 4 g	16 %
Sugars 9 g	
Protein 36 g	
Vitamin A 28 %	Vitamin C 22 %
Calcium 20 %	Iron 40 %
Vitamin K 36 mcg	
Potassium 954 mg	
Magnesium 113 mg	

Fettuccine with Dill Pesto and Shrimp

2 **30 min.**

Serving size = 2 ounces pasta

This recipe requires Dill Pesto be made first (recipe included). This recipe will keep fairly well for a day or so.

4 ounces	fettuccine
4 quarts	water
1 tsp.	extra virgin olive oil
6 ounces	fresh shrimp (peeled and deveined)
2 Tbsp.	dill pesto
1/4 cup	chicken stock
4 ounces	white asparagus spears (steamed)
1/2 ounce	Parmigiano-Reggiano (grated)

Heat the water over high heat in a large stock-pot until boiling. Add the fettuccine.

Place the asparagus in a steamer and as the pasta nears being done (about ten minutes) turn the heat on high.

Heat the olive oil in a large non-stick skillet over medium-high heat.

Add the shrimp and cook on one side for about 2 minutes. Turn and reduce the heat to medium-low and cook for another two minutes.

Add the pesto and chicken stock and toss to coat the shrimp well.

Drain the pasta and add to the pan with the shrimp and pesto.

Divide the steamed asparagus between the two pasta bowls. Fill each bowl with 1/2 of the shrimp/pesto/fettuccini and divide the grated Parmigiano-Reggiano evenly over the top of each dish.

"I drive way too fast to worry about cholesterol."
Steven Wright, Comedian

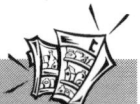

The refrigerator light goes on...
You're not stuck with using basil for your pesto. Almost any green, such as cilantro or arugula, will work. And of course, there's always basil....

Nutrition Facts	
Serving size	2 oz. pasta
Servings	2
Calories 404	Calories from Fat 95
	% Daily Value
Total Fat 11 g	17 %
Saturated Fat 2 g	12 %
Trans Fat 0 g	
Monounsaturated Fat 4 g	
Cholesterol 134 mg	45 %
Sodium 249 mg	10 %
Total Carbohydrates 42 g	14 %
Dietary Fiber 3 g	11 %
Sugars 1 g	
Protein 33 g	
Vitamin A 17 %	Vitamin C 13 %
Calcium 0 %	Iron 33 %
Vitamin K 25 mcg	
Potassium 454 mg	
Magnesium 85 mg	

Meatloaf

6 **75 min.**

Serving size = 6 slices meatloaf.

This keeps well for about 48 hours in the fridge after being cooked. This recipe requires that Tomato Sauce (recipe included) be made first.

1 lb.	extra lean ground beef
4 ounces	fresh bread crumbs
1 tsp.	dried oregano
1 tsp.	dried basil
1 tsp.	dried rosemary
1 tsp.	dried thyme
1/2 tsp.	salt
1/8 tsp.	fresh ground black pepper
3/4 cup	tomato sauce

Preheat oven to 325°F.

Line an oblong Pyrex dish or large skillet with aluminum foil.

Mix the ground beef together with the bread crumbs, oregano, basil, rosemary, thyme, salt and pepper until well blended.

Roll the mixture into a large ball and then shape into a loaf. Place the loaf in the aluminum foil lined pan. Continue to shape until the loaf is firm by pressing it together.

Place the pan in the oven. Cook for about 30 minutes and top with the marinara sauce. Return to the oven and cook for about 20 minutes until the internal temperature is 150°F. Remove from the oven and let rest for about 5 – 10 minutes before slicing.

"Food is the most primitive form of comfort."
Sheilah Graham, Gossip columnist

The refrigerator light goes on...
Meatloaf, next to Mac and Cheese, may be the ultimate comfort food. It's great out of the oven and I like the tomato sauce topping. Served with mashed potatoes and a side of green beans and you can't help but feel good. As with all recipes that use ground beef, look for extra lean or 93 % lean. If need be, ask the butcher to grind you some from a piece of very well trimmed bottom round.

Bottled tomato sauce or marinara sauce will work well with this recipe. Look for a sauce with as little sodium as possible and 2 grams of fat or less per 1/2 cup serving.

Nutrition Facts	
Serving size	1 slice
Servings	6
Calories 193	Calories from Fat 44
	% Daily Value
Total Fat 5 g	8 %
Saturated Fat 2 g	10 %
Trans Fat 0 g	
Monounsaturated Fat 2 g	
Cholesterol 47 mg	16 %
Sodium 387 mg	16 %
Total Carbohydrates 17 g	6 %
Dietary Fiber 2 g	7 %
Sugars 0 g	
Protein 19 g	
Vitamin A 3 %	Vitamin C 8 %
Calcium 6 %	Iron 19 %
Vitamin K 8 mcg	
Potassium 425 mg	
Magnesium 33 mg	

Roasted Salmon with Red Thai Curry

2 **30 min.**

Serving Size = 4 ounces salmon

This recipe can be halved or multiplied by 2 or 3. Does not keep well but the sauce can be made up to 24 hours in advance. This recipe is great served over steamed napa cabbage but it's fantastic served over Plain Mashed Potatoes (recipe included).

1/2 tsp.	hot red bean paste
1/2 cup	reduced-fat coconut milk
1 Tbsp.	grated lemon peel
1 Tbsp.	Splenda
2 Tbsp.	fresh lime juice
2 Tbsp.	sake
1 tsp.	sesame oil
1/2 lb.	shitake mushrooms (sliced)
2 - 4 oz.	salmon filets
1/4 tsp.	salt
2 Tbsp.	cilantro leaves

Place a large non-stick skillet in the oven and preheat to 450°F.

Mix together the red curry paste, coconut milk, lemon peel, Splenda, lime juice and sake. Whisk until smooth.

When the pan is hot place the sesame oil in and swirl to coat the inside. Add the sliced shitake mushrooms to the pan and return to the oven. Check every 3 minutes or so and shake the pan. After about 10 – 12 minutes the mushrooms will be a roasted brown.

Sprinkle the salt over the flesh side of the salmon. Place the filets in the hot pan flesh side down and return to the oven. Cook for about 4 minutes and turn the skin side down. Add the curry sauce and swirl. Return the pan to the oven and cook for another 4 – 5 minutes for rare. Remove and serve.

"Mother's words of wisdom: 'Answer me! Don't talk with food in your mouth!'"

Erma Bombeck, American Domestic Goddess

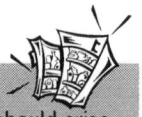

The refrigerator light goes on...
This is another of those recipes that should arise from ingredients in your well stocked pantry. Lemons and limes keep well, cans of coconut milk, sake (or even dry white wine) and your favorite red sauce. After a few weeks of planning it gets easier and easier to cook and eat healthy.

Nutrition Facts	
Serving size	4 oz. salmon
Servings	2
Calories 324	Calories from Fat 166
	% Daily Value
Total Fat 19 g	29 %
Saturated Fat 6 g	29 %
Trans Fat 0 g	
Monounsaturated Fat 5 g	
Cholesterol 66 mg	22 %
Sodium 377 mg	16 %
Total Carbohydrates 9 g	3 %
Dietary Fiber 1 g	4 %
Sugars 4 g	
Protein 25 g	
Vitamin A 3 %	Vitamin C 22 %
Calcium 5 %	Iron 6 %
Vitamin K 4 mcg	
Potassium 956 mg	
Magnesium 45 mg	

Indian Shrimp Curry

4 **30 min.**

Serving size = about 2 cups (4 ounces shrimp)

This recipe can easily be multiplied by 2 or 3. Leftovers are great. Reheat gently.

2 tsp.	extra virgin olive oil
2 cloves	garlic (minced)
1 medium	white onion (sliced)
1 medium	red onion (sliced)
1 cup	2% milk
1 Tbsp.	corn starch
1 Tbsp.	curry powder
2 Tbsp.	honey
1/2 tsp.	salt
1 cup	low-fat (lite) unsweetened coconut milk
1 lb.	large shrimp (peeled and deveined)
4 Tbsp.	fresh cilantro leaves

Heat the olive oil in large non-stick skillet over medium-high heat.

Add the garlic and onion and reduce the heat to medium. Cook gently, stirring frequently, until the onions begin to soften.

While the onions are cooking place the cornstarch in a cup and add 1/4 cup of the 2% milk stirring until the cornstarch is dissolved.

After the onions are soft add the curry powder, honey, salt, lite coconut milk and remaining 2% milk to the skillet. Stir well until the ingredients are well blended and then add the milk/cornstarch mixture.

Reduce the heat to medium-low and cook for about three minutes.

Add shrimp and simmer until they are opaque in center (about 5 minutes).

Serve the curry over Jasmine Rice and top with 1 tablespoon cilantro leaves per serving.

"Some writers say the leaves [cilantro] are used for seasoning, but this statement seems odd, as all the green parts of the plant exhale a very strong odor of the wood-bug, whence the Greek name of the plant."

Vilmorin-Andrieux, author
The Vegetable Garden (1885)

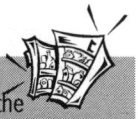

The refrigerator light goes on...
With the discussion of how important the combination of cholesterol and saturated fat are to your health this recipe is an example of how you can make any recipe work for you.

Nutrition Facts	
Serving size	about 2 cups
Servings	4
Calories 272	Calories from Fat 84
	% Daily Value
Total Fat 10 g	15 %
Saturated Fat 5 g	25 %
Trans Fat 0 g	
Monounsaturated Fat 3 g	
Cholesterol 175 mg	58 %
Sodium 499 mg	21 %
Total Carbohydrates 20 g	7 %
Dietary Fiber 1 g	5 %
Sugars 14 g	
Protein 26 g	
Vitamin A 6 %	Vitamin C 12 %
Calcium 17 %	Iron 22 %
Vitamin K 6 mcg	
Potassium 457 mg	
Magnesium 69 mg	

Mushroom Risotto

3 **45 min.**

Serving size = about 2 cups

This recipe is easily multiplied by 2. This keeps well for a few days in the refrigerator.

1 tsp.	extra virgin olive oil
3 cloves	garlic (minced)
1 small	white onion (minced)
1/4 lb.	button mushrooms (sliced)
1 cups	arborio rice
1/4 cup	white wine
2 cups	water
1/8 tsp.	salt
	black pepper (to taste)
2 oz.	wild mushrooms (morels, shiitake or oyster)
1 Tbsp. (per serving)	fresh basil
1 1/2 oz.	Parmigiano-Reggiano
2	medium tomatoes (seeded and julienned)

Heat the olive oil over medium-heat in a medium sized stock-pot. Add the minced garlic and cook slowly. Do not allow to brown.

When the garlic is soft and translucent, add the onions and cook until they are also translucent. Add the button mushrooms and cook over medium-high heat until they begin to turn brown. Continue to cook, stirring continuously until the mushrooms are a dark roasted brown.

Add the risotto and cook for about 2 minutes, stirring frequently.

Reduce the heat to medium and add the white wine .Stir well. Cook for one minute and add 2 cups of water, the salt and pepper.

Cook over medium-heat, stirring frequently so that the rice will not stick to the bottom. After about 15 minutes, check to see if the rice is done. Add more water, 1/4 cup at a time as needed.

Slice the wild mushrooms.

When the rice is soft but not mushy, add the basil, wild mushrooms and parmesan cheese. Stir and cook for another 2 - 3 minutes over very low heat.

Serve topped with the julienne tomatoes.

"We are indeed much more than what we eat, but what we eat can nevertheless help us to be much more than what we are."

Adelle Davis, Nutritionist

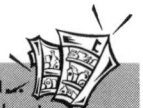

The refrigerator light goes on...
Cooking mushrooms is not a timid enterprise. Because they are mostly water, mushrooms must be cooked until they begin to caramelize to bring out their rich flavor.

Nutrition Facts	
Serving size	about 2 cups
Servings	6
Calories 345	Calories from Fat 63
	% Daily Value
Total Fat 7 g	9 %
Saturated Fat 3 g	15 %
Trans Fat 0 g	
Monounsaturated Fat 0 g	
Cholesterol 0 mg	4 %
Sodium 372 mg	15 %
Total Carbohydrates 59 g	20 %
Dietary Fiber 3 g	11 %
Sugars 0 g	
Protein 12 g	
Vitamin A 10 %	Vitamin C 15 %
Calcium 28 %	Iron 15 %
Vitamin K 19 mcg	
Potassium 585 mg	
Magnesium 2 mg	

Roasted Salmon and Corn Relish

2 **30 min.**

Serving size = 1 - 4 ounce salmon filet with relish

This recipe can easily be multiplied by 2 or 3. Leftovers are great. I like to make sandwiches from the salmon and relish but both go well chilled on top of salads.

Relish	
1	red bell pepper
1/2 tsp.	grapeseed oil
1 cup (~ 1 ear)	fresh corn kernels
1 Tbsp. (~ 1 small)	shallot (minced)
1 small clove	garlic (minced)
1 1/2 tsp.	fresh thyme leaves
2 Tbsp.	dry white wine
1 1/2 tsp.	fresh lime juice
1 1/2 tsp.	honey
1/8 tsp	salt
Sauce	
1 1/2 tsp.	grapeseed oil
1 Tbsp.	fresh lime juice
1 1/2 tsp.	honey
1 1/2 tsp.	paprika
1/8 tsp.	salt
Fish	
2 (4 oz.)	salmon filets
1 tsp.	fresh cilantro (chopped)

Preheat oven to broil. Place the pepper in the oven and char, turning about every 3 minutes until black on all sides. Remove and place in a paper bag.

After about ten to twenty minutes remove peppers from bag. Peel, seed and set aside 1/2 of the pepper in the refrigerator for later. Cut the remaining pepper into 1/2-inch pieces.

Slice the white part of the green onion separate from the green tops.

Heat the grapeseed oil in heavy large non-stick skillet over medium-high heat. Add the corn, the white part of the green onions, the shallot and the garlic. Sauté gently until the corn begins to brown.

Add the thyme and white wine. Cook over low heat until the wine evaporates.

Stir in bell peppers, lime juice, honey, salt, the green tops of the green onions and parsley. Remove from heat. The relish can be made up to 24 hours in advance and reheated gently while the salmon is roasting.

Stir together the 1 Tbsp. grapeseed oil, lime juice, honey, paprika and salt. The sauce can be made up to 24 hours in advance.

When ready to serve preheat oven to 400°F. Line a roasting pan or skillet with foil. Place salmon in middle and top with the sauce. Place in the hot oven and roast for about ten minutes. While the salmon is roasting, gently reheat the corn relish. After ten minutes of roasting, remove the salmon and top each filet with 1/4 of the relish and garnish with fresh cilantro.

The refrigerator light goes on...
The amount of calories seems like a lot for a single entrée but this includes the corn relish, which is a starch, and there are plenty of vegetables. Pair this with a simple salad and you have the perfect meal for a dinner party.

Nutrition Facts	
Serving size	4 oz. salmon w/relish
Servings	4
Calories 368	Calories from Fat 137
	% Daily Value
Total Fat 15 g	24 %
Saturated Fat 2 g	11 %
Trans Fat 0 g	
Monounsaturated Fat 6 g	
Cholesterol 70 mg	23 %
Sodium 359 mg	15 %
Total Carbohydrates 31 g	10 %
Dietary Fiber 4 g	14 %
Sugars 14 g	
Protein 27 g	
Vitamin A 60 %	Vitamin C 143 %
Calcium 3 %	Iron 10 %
Vitamin K 6 mcg	
Potassium 804 mg	
Magnesium 61 mg	

Corn Quesadillas

2 **30 min.**

Serving size = 1 quesadilla

This recipe can easily be multiplied by 2, 3 or 4. Leftovers are sort of like cold pizza (an acquired taste).

1/2 tsp.	grapeseed oil
1/4	poblano chili (seeded and diced)
1 ear	corn (shave kernels from the cob)
1/2 medium	red bell pepper (seeded and julienned)
1/4 tsp.	ground cumin
1/8 tsp.	salt
1 Tbsp.	cilantro leaf (chopped)
	spray oil
4	reduced-fat corn tortillas
2 oz.	reduced-fat Monterey jack cheese (shredded)

Heat the grapeseed oil in a large non-stick skillet over medium heat and add the chili. Cook for about 3 - 5 minutes until soft.

Add the corn and increase the heat to medium-high. Cook the corn kernels, tossing frequently, until they begin to brown.

Add the green onions and cook for about 3 minutes.

Add the red pepper, cumin and salt and cook for 5 minutes until the red pepper begins to soften.

Turn off the heat and add the cilantro and toss until blended into the vegetable mixture.

Preheat oven to 350°F. Place a large non-stick cookie sheet inside while the oven is preheating. After it is hot, spray the cookie sheet lightly with oil and place 4 flour tortillas on top of the cookie sheet.

Top each tortilla with the 1/4 of the corn mixture and then 1 ounce of shredded Monterey jack cheese.
Place a tortilla on top of the corn and cheese forming the quesadilla. Spray very lightly with oil. Return the cookie sheet to the oven and turn on the broiler.

Cook for about 3 – 5 minutes on each side. Turn at least once.

"Sex is good, but not as good as fresh sweet corn."
Garrison Keillor, American humorist

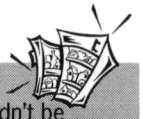

The refrigerator light goes on...
This is one of those recipes that wouldn't be possible without a non-stick pan and spray oil. The quesadillas that you get at Mexican restaurants are greasy because they use so much oil on the griddle (and no one is really paying attention to your arteries).

Nutrition Facts	
Serving size	1 Quesadilla
Servings	2
Calories 273	Calories from Fat 83
	% Daily Value
Total Fat 9 g	14 %
Saturated Fat 4 g	22 %
Trans Fat 0 g	
Monounsaturated Fat 2 g	
Cholesterol 18 mg	6 %
Sodium 345 mg	14 %
Total Carbohydrates 37 g	12 %
Dietary Fiber 6 g	22 %
Sugars 4 g	
Protein 13 g	
Vitamin A 32 %	Vitamin C 92 %
Calcium 25 %	Iron 9 %
Vitamin K 25 mcg	
Potassium 370 mg	
Magnesium 66 mg	

Jerk Shrimp

2 **30 min.**

Serving size = 4 ounces shrimp and 1/4 cup melon salsa

This recipe can easily be multiplied by 2, 3 or 4. Leftovers are great in sandwiches and salads. The Jerk Seasoning Blend needs to be made beforehand.

Serve with Mango or Melon Salsa (recipe included), lime wedges, and Coconut Rice (recipe included).

8 oz.	large shrimp (peeled & deveined)
2 tsp.	grapeseed oil or canola oil
1 Tbsp.	fresh lime juice
2 tsp.	jerk seasoning blend
2	lime wedges
1/2 cup	melon salsa
1 Tbsp.	cilantro leaves

Prepare the barbecue (medium heat) if the jerk is to be grilled. If using a grill pan instead of using a grill, preheat oven to 400°F and place the grill pan inside.

Place the shrimp, grapeseed oil, lime juice and jerk seasoning blend in medium bowl. Let marinate at least ten minutes.

Thread shrimp onto metal or soaked wooden skewers.

Grill on the barbecue or grill pan for about 2 minutes on the first side and then turn. Cook until opaque in the center. Brush frequently with marinade. Total cooking time will be about 5 - 7 minutes.

"Pepper is small in quantity and great in virtue."
Plato

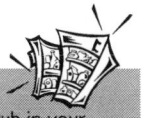

The refrigerator light goes on...
Bang, bang you're done. Keep some jerk rub in your spice cabinet and you can toss it on shrimp or chicken breasts. A little sweet salsa is easy to make and in 20 minutes you are ready to put on some Jimmy Buffett and chow down.

Nutrition Facts	
Serving size	4 oz. shrimp with 1/4 cup salsa
Servings	2
Calories 185	Calories from Fat 59
	% Daily Value
Total Fat 7 g	10 %
Saturated Fat 1 g	4 %
Trans Fat 0 g	
Monounsaturated Fat 1 g	
Cholesterol 173 mg	57 %
Sodium 314 mg	13 %
Total Carbohydrates 8 g	3 %
Dietary Fiber 1 g	4 %
Sugars 4 g	
Protein 23 g	
Vitamin A 23 %	Vitamin C 27 %
Calcium 8 %	Iron 19 %
Vitamin K 6 mcg	
Potassium 357 mg	
Magnesium 51 mg	

Jerk Rub

Servings = 24
Serving size = 1 teaspoon
Makes 1/2 cup

Keeps very well for months sealed tightly.

1 small	dried chipotle
1 Tbsp.	black peppercorns
1 Tbsp.	onion powder
2 tsp.	allspice
2 tsp.	cinnamon
1/2 tsp..	ground cumin
1 Tbsp	coriander seeds
1 Tbsp.	garlic powder
1 Tbsp.	ground ginger
1 Tbsp.	thyme
1/2 tsp.	ground nutmeg
1 Tbsp.	light brown sugar
1/2 tsp.	whole cloves
1 tsp..	salt

Combine all ingredients in a blender and blend on high speed until all ingredients are powdered.

"The joys of the table belong equally to all ages, conditions, countries and times; they mix with all other pleasures, and remain the last to console us for their loss."

Jean-Anthelme Brillat-Savarin, Gourmond

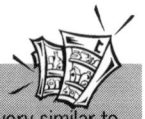

The refrigerator light goes on...
There are a lot of dry rubs on the market very similar to this jerk. There's essentially nothing in them but flavor so you can use almost as much as your spicy palate will allow. Many do have more salt in them than this recipe so check the Nutrition Facts carefully.

Nutrition Facts	
Serving size	1 teaspoon
Servings	24
Calories 8	Calories from Fat 0
	% Daily Value
Total Fat 0 g	0 %
Saturated Fat 0 g	0 %
Trans Fat 0 g	
Monounsaturated Fat 0 g	
Cholesterol 0 mg	0 %
Sodium 98 mg	4 %
Total Carbohydrates 2 g	1 %
Dietary Fiber 0 g	2 %
Sugars 1 g	
Protein 0 g	
Vitamin 0 7 %	Vitamin C 1 %
Calcium 1 %	Iron 2 %
Vitamin K 2 mcg	
Potassium 0 mg	
Magnesium 0 mg	

Chicken with Tarragon Mustard Cream

2 **30 min.**

Serving size = 4 ounces chicken breast

This recipe can easily be multiplied by 2 or 3. Leftovers are fair at best.

1 tsp.	extra virgin olive oil
2 – 4 oz.	boneless, skinless chicken breasts
1/2 cup	chicken stock
2 oz.	goat cheese
2 tsp.	coarse ground mustard
1/4 cup	2% milk
1/8 tsp.	dried tarragon

Preheat oven to 300°F.

Heat oil in a large non-stick skillet over medium high heat. Add chicken breasts and allow to cook for about 2 - 3 minutes, without turning. Then turn and cook for 2 minutes. (The surface should be seared brown on both sides.)

Remove the chicken and place on a sheet of foil to catch any juices and put in the preheated oven.

Deglaze the pan with the chicken stock and allow the sauce to reduce by about half.

Remove from the heat and add the goat cheese. Whisk in the cheese with the pan off of the heat until the sauce is smooth.

With the pan still off of the heat, add the mustard, milk and tarragon. Stir until the sauce is smooth.

Reduce the heat to low-medium and place the pan back on the burner. As the sauce slowly reheats remove the chicken breasts from the oven and place in the sauce. Turn frequently as the sauce and chicken breasts heat through (they are ready when the internal temperature is 160°F).

"No diet will remove all the fat from your body because the brain is entirely fat. Without a brain you might look good, but all you could do is run for public office."

Covert Bailey, 1980s fitness guru

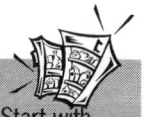

The refrigerator light goes on...
Rich, creamy sauces can be healthy. Start with less fat, cooking the roux carefully, stir constantly when adding the liquid and thicken with a lower fat creamy cheese.

Nutrition Facts	
Serving size	4 oz. chicken
Servings	2
Calories 271	Calories from Fat 114
	% Daily Value
Total Fat 13 g	20 %
Saturated Fat 7 g	35 %
Trans Fat 0 g	
Monounsaturated Fat 4 g	
Cholesterol 91 mg	30 %
Sodium 418 mg	17 %
Total Carbohydrates 3 g	1 %
Dietary Fiber 0 g	1 %
Sugars 3 g	
Protein 34 g	
Vitamin A 9 %	Vitamin C 3 %
Calcium 15 %	Iron 8 %
Vitamin K 2 mcg	
Potassium 409 mg	
Magnesium 47 mg	

Halibut with Seven Spices

2 **30 min.**

Serving size = 4 ounces fish

This recipe can easily be multiplied by 2 or 3. Serve with Rice and Lentil Pilaf (recipe included; make first). The fish makes good leftovers for sandwiches or salads.

1 tsp.	extra virgin olive oil
1 Tbsp.	pine nuts
2 Tbsp.	capers
1 large	tomato (seeded and sliced into julienne strips)
1/8 tsp.	salt
2 Tbsp.	balsamic vinegar
to taste	fresh ground black pepper
1 tsp.	unsalted butter
2 - 4 oz.	halibut filets (without skin)
1/8 tsp.	seven spice seasoning
	spray olive oil

Preheat the oven to 400°F. Place a medium or large skillet in the oven.

Place the olive oil in a medium non-stick skillet over medium-low heat. Add the pine nuts, capers and tomato and cook for about 2 minutes stirring once. Add salt, balsamic vinegar, pepper and butter and reduce the heat to low. Stir occasionally.

Sprinkle the halibut filets with seven spice seasoning.

Spray the hot pan from the oven lightly with olive oil and place the halibut filets in the hot pan seasoned side down. Return the pan to the oven and cook for about 4 - 5 minutes. Turn the filets and cook for another 4 - 5 minutes depending on thickness.

Remove and serve on top of Rice and Lentil Pilaf. Top with the tomato caper mixture.

Suhtain ~ The Lebanese word for "enjoy this food in good health."

The refrigerator light goes on...
This recipe is a great example of one that is higher in fat but low in saturated fat. While I try to keep Dr. Gourmet recipes under 15 grams of fat per serving, keep in mind that it is your average intake that is important. One day you might eat more and other days less. It is the long term reduction of fat, calories and cholesterol that can help you live longer and live better.

Those recipes that are higher in fat are like this one and have high levels of the healthy fats like monounsaturated fats and Omega 3 fats.

Seven spice seasoning is the best. Every time I open the spice drawer that I keep my ziplock bag full of this pungent spice in, the aroma evokes the market place and a spice merchant doling out small bags of spices. The market is crowded and loud with the bartering sellers and buyers. (Mind you, I've never been to such a place but the fragrance for the spice is so heady I feel that I know it.)

Nutrition Facts	
Serving size	4 oz. fish
Servings	2
Calories 229	Calories from Fat 103
	% Daily Value
Total Fat 12 g	18 %
Saturated Fat 2 g	11 %
Trans Fat 0 g	
Monounsaturated Fat 4 g	
Cholesterol 41 mg	14 %
Sodium 469 mg	20 %
Total Carbohydrates 5 g	2 %
Dietary Fiber 2 g	7 %
Sugars 5 g	
Protein 25 g	
Vitamin A 20 %	Vitamin C 20 %
Calcium 7 %	Iron 10 %
Vitamin K 15 mcg	
Potassium 777 mg	
Magnesium 124 mg	

Mojo Pork Tenderloin

4 **60 min.**

Serving size = 4 ounces pork

This recipe can easily be halved or multiplied by 2. Leftovers are great for sandwiches.

2	navel oranges (juiced)
1	lime (juiced)
1 Tbsp	flat leaf parsley (chopped fine)
1 Tbsp.	fresh oregano (chopped fine)
1 tsp.	fresh thyme leaves
1 cloves	garlic (minced)
1/4 tsp.	salt
1 Tbsp.	extra virgin olive oil
16 oz. (1 large)	pork tenderloin (well trimmed)

Mix together the orange juice, lime juice, chopped parsley, chopped oregano, thyme leaves, minced garlic, salt and olive oil in a large glass bowl. (This makes approximately 3 cups.)

Place the pork tenderloins in a zipper bag and add two cups of the marinade. Seal the bag and marinate at least overnight. Place the remaining marinade in the refrigerator.

When you are ready to cook the pork, place a large non-stick skillet in an oven and preheat to 450°F.

While the pan is preheating, remove the marinating pork tenderloin and the extra marinade. Strain the cup of extra marinade in a small sauce pan over high heat and bring to a boil. Reduce the heat to medium and simmer gently to reduce by half.

Remove the pork tenderloins and place them on a plate. Strain the remaining marinade and discard the strained herbs and garlic, reserving the liquid.

Place the pork tenderloins in the preheated pan and return the pan to the oven. Cook for about 4 minutes and turn the pork every 3 minutes after that, until all the sides are seared. After the second turn, baste with 1/2 cup of the strained marinade, coating the tenderloins well.
As the pork cooks and the marinade is reduced, continue to baste with 1/4 to 1/2 cup at a time to create a caramelized glaze on the pork. It should take 20 – 25 minutes to reach an internal temperature of 160°F.

As the pork is finishing, add the remaining marinade to create a syrupy sauce.

Remove the pork from the oven and let rest on the counter for about 3 minutes before carving. Serve with the reduced sauce from the pan.

"We must eat to live and live to eat."
Henry Fielding, Author

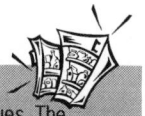

The refrigerator light goes on...
This recipe has so many valuable techniques. The marinade tenderizes and adds flavor while keeping food juicy. Braising is key to moist juicy meats. While this recipe uses a tender cut to begin with, tougher cuts of meat turn out well when braised. Basting helps create a rich glaze and the marinade makes a rich tangy sauce by slow reduction. All perfect over mashed potatoes.

Nutrition Facts	
Serving size	4 oz. pork w/sauce
Servings	4
Calories 185	Calories from Fat 53
	% Daily Value
Total Fat 6 g	9 %
Saturated Fat 1 g	6 %
Trans Fat 0 g	
Monounsaturated Fat 4 g	
Cholesterol 73 mg	24 %
Sodium 206 mg	9 %
Total Carbohydrates 8 g	3 %
Dietary Fiber 0 g	2 %
Sugars 0 g	
Protein 24 g	
Vitamin A 3 %	Vitamin C 42 %
Calcium 2 %	Iron 10 %
Vitamin K 23 mcg	
Potassium 592 mg	
Magnesium 40 mg	

Tomato Saffron Risotto with Salmon

2 **30 min.**

Serving size = about 2 cups

This recipe can easily be multiplied by 2 or 3. This keeps well for about 48 hours in the fridge. Reheat gently.

1 cup	water
1 ounce	sun-dried tomatoes
1 tsp.	olive oil
2 cloves	garlic (minced)
1 large	shallot (diced)
1 large	leek (sliced)
1/2 cup	arborio rice
4 cups	water
1/4 tsp.	salt
1/8 tsp.	fresh ground black pepper
10 threads	saffron
1 oz.	Parmigiano-Reggiano (grated)
8 oz.	salmon filet (skinless, cut into 1/2 inch thick strips)

Heat the water in a small sauce pan. When the water is boiling add the sun-dried tomatoes and reduce the heat to a simmer. Let the tomatoes simmer for about ten minutes until soft. About have the liquid will remain. Remove and let stand. When cool puree in a mini chopper or blender.

Heat the olive oil in a large sauce pan over medium heat. Add the garlic and the green tops of the sliced leek. Cook over medium-low heat until the leeks begin to wilt. Add the shallot and the remaining leek.

Stir occasionally and after about 5 minutes add the rice. Stir for about one minute. Strain the liquid from the tomatoes into the pan and stir.

While the rice is cooking over medium-low heat place the sun-dried tomatoes in a blender or a mini chopper. Add 1/4 cup water and puree until a smooth paste.

Add more water to the rice as it cooks and evaporates. Stir occasionally. Add the salt, pepper and saffron. Continue to cook, stirring continuously and adding water gradually. Add the grated Parmigiano-Reggiano and stir until melted.

Taste the rice frequently checking for doneness. For this saffron risotto there should be more liquid and when the rice is stirred there should be about an extra cup of liquid. Add the flaked salmon to the risotto and stir gently for about 3 minutes and serve.

"...saffron, the most aristocratic spice..."
John Humphries, Author, Importer

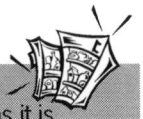

The refrigerator light goes on...
You can eat leftover salmon as long as it is cooked carefully. By cooking the salmon gently at the end of the recipe it won't be overcooked when the leftovers are reheated. Cook the leftover risotto very gently by heating on medium heat in the microwave for 90 seconds. Stir gently and heat for another 90 to 120 seconds until hot.

Nutrition Facts	
Serving size	2 cups
Servings	2
Calories 536	Calories from Fat 172
	% Daily Value
Total Fat 19 g	30 %
Saturated Fat 5 g	27 %
Trans Fat 0 g	
Monounsaturated Fat 7 g	
Cholesterol 78 mg	26 %
Sodium 875 mg	36 %
Total Carbohydrates 56 g	19 %
Dietary Fiber 4 g	16 %
Sugars 7 g	
Protein 34 g	
Vitamin A 21 %	Vitamin C 28 %
Calcium 22 %	Iron 28 %
Vitamin K 29 mcg	
Potassium 1052 mg	
Magnesium 92 mg	

Oven Fried Chicken

4 **30 min.**

Serving size = 1 chicken piece

This recipe can easily be multiplied by 2, 3 or 4. Leftovers keep well for 2 days. Allow to cool before refrigerating.

1	large egg
1	large egg white
1 Tbsp.	Dijon mustard
1 box (5 oz.)	plain melba toast
1 tsp.	dried thyme
1 tsp.	dried rosemary
1/2 tsp.	dried oregano
1/4 tsp.	garlic powder
1/4 tsp.	salt
1/2 tsp.	ground black pepper
1/4 tsp.	cayenne pepper
4 - 4 oz.	boneless, skinless chicken breasts
	spray oil

Place the egg, egg white and Dijon mustard in a small bowl. Whisk until smooth.

In a food processor fitted with a steel blade, place the melba toast, thyme, rosemary, oregano, garlic powder, salt, black pepper and cayenne pepper. Process until small breadcrumbs. Leave some pieces about the size of currants.

Preheat oven to 400°F.

Dredge a chicken breast in the egg mixture, coating thoroughly. Dredge in the breadcrumbs, patting and turning frequently until well coated.

Place the chicken on a cookie sheet or baking rack and then place in oven. Bake for 3 minutes and then lightly spray the top of each chicken breast with the oil. Bake 5 minutes more and then turn. Spray lightly with the oil again and bake for about 6 more minutes.

This recipe works well with any piece of chicken (with or without the bone). Use skinless legs, thighs or breasts.

"It's finger lickin' good."

Col. Harland Sanders,
Founder, Kentucky Fried Chicken

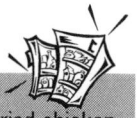

The refrigerator light goes on...
Melba toast is amazing as breading! Fried chicken doesn't have to be fried to taste like fried chicken.

Nutrition Facts	
Serving size	1 chicken breast
Servings	4
Calories 293	Calories from Fat 36
	% Daily Value
Total Fat 4 g	6 %
Saturated Fat 1 g	5 %
Trans Fat 0 g	
Monounsaturated Fat 1 g	
Cholesterol 119 mg	40 %
Sodium 588 mg	25 %
Total Carbohydrates 28 g	9 %
Dietary Fiber 3 g	11 %
Sugars 1 g	
Protein 33 g	
Vitamin A 3 %	Vitamin C 3 %
Calcium 7 %	Iron 16 %
Vitamin K 6 mcg	
Potassium 412 mg	
Magnesium 59 mg	

Chili Rellenos

2 **60 min.**

Serving size = 2 peppers

This recipe can easily be multiplied by 2. Does not keep well.

1 small	dried chipotle chili
1 tsp.	grapeseed oil
1 medium	white onion (minced)
1/4 tsp.	ground cumin
4 medium	poblano peppers
3 oz.	reduced-fat Monterey jack cheese (shredded)
4 Tbsp.	fresh cilantro
1	large egg
1	large egg white
1 Tbsp.	Dijon mustard
4 oz.	plain melba toast
1/4 tsp.	ground cumin
1/4 tsp.	salt
1/4 tsp.	ground black pepper
1/8 tsp.	cayenne pepper

Place a steamer basket in a small sauce pan with about a cup of water in the bottom of it. Heat the steamer over high heat and place the chipotle inside. When it is soft, move it to a cutting board and carefully remove the seeds. Avoid touching the pepper with your hands. If you do, wash them well.

Mince the chipotle and set aside.

Place the canola oil in a large non-stick skillet and heat over medium heat. Add the onion and cook slowly until translucent. Add the minced chipotle and cook for another two minutes. Remove from the heat and chill in the refrigerator for about an hour.
Preheat oven to broil. Place the poblano peppers in the oven and roast them, turning by 1/4 turn about every three minutes. The skin of the chili should begin to turn black. After the skin is blackened, remove the peppers from the oven and place in a brown paper bag.

After about 30 minutes, the peppers should be cool. Remove them from the paper bag and gently peel the thin skin from the pepper. Using the point of a knife, make a slit down the long side of each pepper. Gently remove the core and seeds from the inside, trying to keep the pepper whole.

After the cooked onion is cool, toss it together with the cilantro and shredded cheese. Form the cheese into 8 small cylinders. Place the cylinders inside the peppers and reform the poblanos to resemble whole peppers.

Place the egg, egg white and mustard in a small bowl. Whisk until smooth.

In a food processor, place the melba toast, ground cumin, salt, black pepper and cayenne pepper and process until small bread crumbs. Leave some pieces about the size of currants.

Preheat oven to 400°F.

Coat the peppers with the egg and mustard mixture and then coat with the melba toast crumbs. After all of them are coated, place on a non-stick cookie sheet then put them into the oven. Bake for about 15 minutes. Spray lightly with spray oil and turn at about 7 minutes.

Nutrition Facts	
Serving size	2 peppers
Servings	2
Calories 484	Calories from Fat 146
	% Daily Value
Total Fat 16 g	25 %
Saturated Fat 7 g	36 %
Trans Fat 0 g	
Monounsaturated Fat 4 g	
Cholesterol 133 mg	34 %
Sodium 695 mg	29 %
Total Carbohydrates 59 g	20 %
Dietary Fiber 8 g	32 %
Sugars 8 g	
Protein 26 g	
Vitamin A 23 %	Vitamin C 214 %
Calcium 41 %	Iron 23 %
Vitamin K 19 mcg	
Potassium 626 mg	
Magnesium 79 mg	

Creamy Mac and Cheese

4 **45 min.**

Serving size = 2 ounces pasta

This recipe can easily be multiplied by 2 or 3. Leftovers are good. Reheat gently after adding 1- Tbsp. of 2 % milk per serving.

4 quarts	water
8 oz.	penne pasta
1/2 of a 4 oz. carton	egg substitute
2 tsp.	cornstarch
1/2 cup	1 % milk (2 % milk will work)
5 oz.	reduced-fat cheddar cheese (grated)
1/8 tsp.	salt
	fresh ground black pepper

Place the water in a medium stock-pot over high heat and bring to a boil. Add the pasta and cook until done. Do not overcook – the pasta should be cooked al dente.

While the pasta is cooking, combine the egg substitute, cornstarch, 1 % milk, reduced-fat cheddar cheese and salt in a small glass mixing bowl.

Place the mixing bowl in the microwave and heat on high in 30-second intervals until hot. Whisk with a fork after each 30-second interval. Do not allow the mixture to get so hot that it boils.

When the pasta is done, drain well and return it to the pot. Add the cheese mixture and mix well until the cheese is completely melted and creamy.

Add fresh ground black pepper to taste and serve immediately.

"They take great pride in making their dinner cost much; I take my pride in making my dinner cost so little."

Henry David Thoreau,
Author

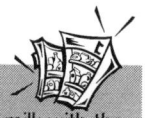

The refrigerator light goes on...
Blending and melting the cheese and milk with the cornstarch first helps to make a creamy sauce.

Nutrition Facts	
Serving size	2 oz. pasta
Servings	2
Calories 304	Calories from Fat 36
	% Daily Value
Total Fat 4 g	6 %
Saturated Fat 2 g	10 %
Trans Fat 0 g	
Monounsaturated Fat 1 g	
Cholesterol 9 mg	3 %
Sodium 340 mg	14 %
Total Carbohydrates 46 g	15 %
Dietary Fiber 2 g	7 %
Sugars 1 g	
Protein 19 g	
Vitamin A 4 %	Vitamin C 1 %
Calcium 21 %	Iron 14 %
Vitamin K 0 mcg	
Potassium 218 mg	
Magnesium 42 mg	

Thai Coconut Shrimp

4 **30 min.**

Serving size = 4 ounces shrimp and 2 tablespoons peanut sauce

This recipe can easily be multiplied by 2, 3 or 4. Leftovers are great. Keeps well for 24 – 36 hours. Serve over Coconut Rice (recipe included) with 2 tablespoons of Thai Peanut sauce (recipe included).`

1/2 cup	light coconut milk
2 cloves	garlic (minced)
2 Tbsp.	fresh lime juice
1 Tbsp.	fresh ginger (peeled & minced)
1 Tbsp.	low-sodium soy sauce
1 tsp.	hoisin sauce
1 Tbsp.	maple syrup
1 cup	Thai basil (finely chopped)
16 oz.	shrimp (peeled and deveined)

Place the low-fat coconut milk, minced garlic, lime juice, minced ginger, low-sodium soy sauce, maple syrup and Thai basil in a blender and puree until smooth.

Using two medium sized wooden skewers assemble small kabobs of shrimp. The amount of shrimp on each kabob will be determined by the size of shrimp that is used. For medium sized shrimp this will be about 4 shrimp per kabob for a total of 8 kabobs.

Put the shrimp in the bottom of an oblong Pyrex dish and add the marinade. Cover tightly with plastic wrap and place in the refrigerator for at least 3 hours (overnight is best).

When ready to cook preheat the oven to 400°F. Place a non-stick grill pan or skillet in the oven and let heat for at least 10 minutes. When hot add the marinated shrimp skewers. As they sear on one side top the other with about half of the marinade.

The shrimp will grill fast and should be turned after about three minutes. Spread the remaining marinade over the top of the shrimp and grill for another 4 – 5 minutes.

"Pounding fragrant things, particularly garlic, basil, parsley, is a tremendous antidote to depression."

Patience Gray, Author and artist

The refrigerator light goes on...
Shrimp has very few calories and almost no fat. While it does have a lot of cholesterol by comparison to other foods, if you are careful to not combine it with too much saturated fat, the shrimp dishes that you know and love can become part of your diet with no problem.

Nutrition Facts	
Serving size	4 oz. shrimp w/2 Tbsp. peanut sauce
Servings	8
Calories 173	Calories from Fat 45
	% Daily Value
Total Fat 5 g	8 %
Saturated Fat 3 g	16 %
Trans Fat 0 g	
Monounsaturated Fat 0 g	
Cholesterol 170 mg	57 %
Sodium 340 mg	14 %
Total Carbohydrates 7 g	2 %
Dietary Fiber 0 g	1 %
Sugars 4 g	
Protein 24 g	
Vitamin A 10 %	Vitamin C 11 %
Calcium 8 %	Iron 20 %
Vitamin K 25 mcg	
Potassium 299 mg	
Magnesium 56 mg	

Salmon with Parmesan Crust

2 **30 min.**

Serving size = 4 ounces salmon filet

This recipe can be multiplied easily by 2, 3 or 4. The bread crumb mixture will keep well overnight tightly covered.

2 oz.	fresh sourdough bread
1 ounce	Parmigiano-Reggiano (grated)
1 small clove	garlic (minced)
1 Tbsp.	fresh basil (chiffonade)
1 Tsp.	extra virgin olive oil
1/2 Tbsp.	balsamic vinegar
2 – 4 oz.	salmon filets (no more than 1/2 in. thick)
	spray olive oil

Add the fresh sourdough bread to a food processor and process until they are fine crumbs.

Add the parmesan, garlic, basil, olive oil and vinegar and process until the mixture is well combined. This will make a moist breadcrumb mixture.

Preheat the oven to 450°. Place a non-stick skillet in the oven on the lowest possible rack. Remove the middle rack. Leave the pan in the oven for at least ten minutes.

Place the salmon fillets on a cutting board skin side down and pat the breadcrumb mixture onto the top of each fillet.

Remove the skillet from the oven and lightly spray with oil. Transfer the salmon filets (skin side down) to the pan and return to the oven. Cook for 6 minutes for rare.

Switch on the broiler and broil until the crust is golden brown (about 3 - 5 more minutes).

"Find something you're passionate about and keep tremendously interested in it."

Julia Child, Pioneer

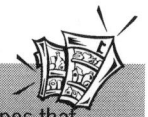

The refrigerator light goes on...
This is one of a series of salmon recipes that are all quick and simple recipes and rely on ingredients that you should already have in the house. And you don't have to use salmon. Any fish with some character will hold up to these recipes.

Nutrition Facts	
Serving size	1 salmon filet
Servings	2
Calories 394	Calories from Fat 190
	% Daily Value
Total Fat 21 g	33 %
Saturated Fat 5 g	26 %
Trans Fat 0 g	
Monounsaturated Fat 11 g	
Cholesterol 83 mg	28 %
Sodium 445 mg	19 %
Total Carbohydrates 16 g	5 %
Dietary Fiber 1 g	4 %
Sugars 1 g	
Protein 30 g	
Vitamin A 7 %	Vitamin C 1 %
Calcium 19 %	Iron 8 %
Vitamin K 10 mcg	
Potassium 504 mg	
Magnesium 42 mg	

Fettuccine Alfredo

2 **30 min.**

Serving size = 2 ounces pasta with sauce

This recipe can easily be multiplied by 2, 3 or 4. Leftovers are fair at best.

1 tsp.	extra virgin olive oil
2 cloves	roasted garlic
2 tsp.	all purpose white flour
3/4 cup	2 % milk
1 ounce	semi-soft goat cheese
1 ounce	Parmigiano-Reggiano (grated)
4 quarts	water
4 ounces	whole wheat fettuccine
1 Tbsp.	fresh Italian or curly parsley (minced)

Heat the olive oil in a ten-inch non-stick skillet over medium heat and add the minced garlic. Cook very slowly and stir frequently. Do not allow the garlic to brown or it will become bitter.

Add the flour slowly and cook for about one minute. Stir continuously to blend the oil and flour. The mixture will be like coarse corn meal. Cook gently so the mixture doesn't brown.

Slowly add the cold milk whisking to keep the sauce from forming clumps. Blend in all of the milk until the sauce is smooth and begins to thicken.

Add the goat cheese and whisk as it melts. When the sauce is smooth add the Parmigiano-Reggiano and whisk as it melts until the sauce is creamy. Reduce the heat to very low.

In a large pot heat the water to a boil. Add the fettuccine and cook until just tender (about 12 – 15 minutes for dried pasta). Drain well and then add the pasta to the sauce tossing to coat thoroughly. Sprinkle the minced parsley over the top and serve.

"Tomatoes and oregano make it Italian; wine and tarragon make it French. Sour cream makes it Russian; lemon and cinnamon make it Greek. Soy sauce makes it Chinese; garlic makes it good."

Alice May Brock, Owner
of Alice's Restaurant

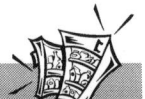

The refrigerator light goes on...
Rich, creamy sauces can be healthy. Start with less fat, cooking the roux carefully, stir constantly when adding the liquid and thicken with a lower fat creamy cheese.

Nutrition Facts	
Serving size	2 oz. pasta
Servings	2
Calories 389	Calories from Fat 107
	% Daily Value
Total Fat 12 g	19 %
Saturated Fat 6 g	30 %
Trans Fat 0 g	
Monounsaturated Fat 5 g	
Cholesterol 23 mg	8 %
Sodium 337 mg	14 %
Total Carbohydrates 53 g	18 %
Dietary Fiber 5 g	20 %
Sugars 5 g	
Protein 20 g	
Vitamin A 7 %	Vitamin C 11 %
Calcium 36 %	Iron 16 %
Vitamin K 33 mcg	
Potassium 354 mg	
Magnesium 107 mg	

London Broil with Mushroom Sautéed in Cognac

3 **60 min.**

Serving size = 4 oz. steak with about 1/2 cup mushrooms

This recipe is easily multiplied but steaks should be no more than about 1.5 Lbs. Leftovers are great. Serve with Garlic Mashed Potatoes (recipe included).

1 tsp.	extra virgin olive oil
1/2 tsp.	grapeseed oil
3/4 Lbs.	small crimini mushrooms (halved)
1/2 cup	shallot (minced)
3 Tbsp.	Cognac (bourbon will do also)
6 Tbsp.	non-fat beef stock
1 Tbsp.	pure maple syrup
to taste	fresh ground black pepper 1/2
Tbsp.	unsalted butter
1 lb.	lean London broil (top round)
1/8 tsp.	salt
to taste	fresh ground black pepper

Preheat the oven to 400°F.

Place a 12 inch non-stick skillet in the oven for about ten minutes. Remove and add the grapeseed oil to the pan and swirl to coat the pan well. Add the mushrooms and shallots and toss until well blended. Return the pan to the oven. Check the mushrooms about every 5 minutes and toss well. Stir with a wooden spatula, if necessary.

After about 15 minutes, the mushrooms will be well browned. Add the cognac, beef stock, maple syrup, pepper and butter. Toss well and return to the oven. Cook for another ten minutes, to reduce the liquid by about half. Remove the pan and set aside.

Place a 12 inch non-stick grill pan or skillet in the oven at 400°F. Heat for about ten minutes. While it is heating, carefully sprinkle 1/2 of the 1/8 teaspoon of salt across the top of the steak. Grind black pepper across the top. When the grill pan is hot, place the steak in, seasoned side down. Return the grill pan to the oven.
Before turning the steak, sprinkle the remaining salt over the top.

Rare steak takes about 8 minutes of the first side and 6 minutes after the turn. Medium rare steak takes about 12 minutes of the first side and 8 minutes after the turn. Remove the steak from the oven and turn the oven off. Place the pan with the mushrooms back in the oven. Place the steak on a cutting board and allow it to rest for 3 – 5 minutes. When ready to carve, slice the beef very thin cutting across the grain.

Serve over Garlic Mashed Potatoes and top with 1/3 of the sautéed mushrooms.

"Red meat is not bad for you. Now blue-green meat, that's bad for you!"

Tommy Smothers, Confused brother and singer

The refrigerator light goes on...
Eating healthy does not mean that you have to eat chicken or fish all the time.

Nutrition Facts	
Serving size 4 oz. meat w/mushrooms	
Servings	3
Calories 327	Calories from Fat 114
	% Daily Value
Total Fat 13 g	20 %
Saturated Fat 5 g	25 %
Trans Fat 0 g	
Monounsaturated Fat 5 g	
Cholesterol 72 mg	24 %
Sodium 217 mg	9 %
Total Carbohydrates 16 g	5 %
Dietary Fiber 1 g	3 %
Sugars 6 g	
Protein 29 g	
Vitamin A 10 %	Vitamin C 5 %
Calcium 4 %	Iron 18 %
Vitamin K 0 mcg	
Potassium 1075 mg	
Magnesium 47 mg	

Philly Cheese Steak

1 **30 min.**

Serving size = 1 sandwich

This recipe can easily be multiplied. This recipe requires leftovers and should be eaten immediately. This recipe is good using any leftover flank steak or London broil recipe.

	olive oil spray
1/2	medium onion (peeled and sliced)
1	mini baguette (2.5 oz.or less)
1 Tbsp.	non-fat mayonnaise
2 oz.	roasted flank steak or London broil (thinly sliced)
1/2 oz.	reduced-fat Swiss cheese (shredded)

Spray a non-stick pan with olive oil and place over a medium-high heat.

After the pan is hot, add the onions and reduce the heat to medium. Cook the onions slowly until they are well browned. Set aside.

Preheat the oven to broil.

Slice the mini baguette lengthwise and place under the broiler with the cut side of the bread facing up until the inside is slightly brown.

Remove from the oven and spread the mayonnaise on the bread and top with the sliced flank steak Top with the onions and then place the Swiss cheese on top of the sandwich.

Return the sandwich to the oven with the cheese side up and broil until the cheese is hot and melted.

"America is a confirmed sandwich nation. Everywhere you go you find sandwich stands, sandwich shops, and nine out of ten people seem to stick to the sandwich-and-glass-of-milk or cup-of-coffee luncheon."

James Beard, Father of American Cuisine

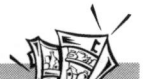

The refrigerator light goes on...
Recipes with flank steak or London Broil make for a wonderful, lean and tasty dinner but here's the bonus – leftovers.

Nutrition Facts	
Serving size	1 sandwich
Servings	1
Calories 395	Calories from Fat 123
	% Daily Value
Total Fat 14 g	21 %
Saturated Fat 4 g	19 %
Trans Fat 0 g	
Monounsaturated Fat 3 g	
Cholesterol 41 mg	14 %
Sodium 524 mg	22 %
Total Carbohydrates 43 g	14 %
Dietary Fiber 6 g	25 %
Sugars 9 g	
Protein 26 g	
Vitamin A 1 %	Vitamin C 8 %
Calcium 23 %	Iron 16 %
Vitamin K 26 mcg	
Potassium 495 mg	
Magnesium 84 mg	

Sea Bass with White Beans and Tomato Vinaigrette

2 **30 min.**

Serving size = 4 ounces fish with beans

This recipe can easily be multiplied by 2 or 3. This recipe does not make very good leftovers.

1 1/2 cups	water
1 oz.	dried wild mushroom (like porcini)
12	grape tomatoes (quartered)
1 Tbsp.	olive oil
1 tsp.	balsamic vinegar
1 tsp.	olive oil
1 slice (about 1 oz.)	prosciutto ham (diced)
1/2 cup	carrot (small dice)
1/2 cup	celery (small dice)
1/2 cup	white part of leek (small dice)
1 - 15 oz. can	white beans (drained and rinsed well)
1/4 tsp.	dried oregano
1/4 tsp.	salt
to taste	fresh ground black pepper
2 - 4 oz. filets	sea bass (or other fatty white fish like halibut)
	spray olive oil

Place the water in a sauce pan over high heat. When the water boils add the dried porcini mushrooms and reduce the heat until the water is simmering. After the stock has cooked for about 15 minutes remove the pan from the heat.

Place the cut tomatoes, 1 Tbsp. olive oil and vinegar in a small bowl and toss well. Place the vinaigrette in the refrigerator to chill.

Preheat the oven to 400°F. Place a large non-stick skillet inside while the oven is preheating.

Place the 1 tsp. olive oil in a medium skillet over medium heat. Add the prosciutto and cook, stirring frequently for about 1 minute.Add the carrot and celery and cook, stirring frequently, for about two minutes. Add the leek and cook for another minute, stirring frequently.

Add the white beans, salt, pepper and oregano. Strain the mushroom broth into the skillet with the white beans and discard the porcini mushrooms.

Reduce the heat to simmer. Stir occasionally while the fish cooks.

Lightly spray the skillet in the oven with olive oil. Add the sea bass skin side down and return to the oven. Cook for about 6 minutes and turn the fish over.

While the fish is cooking divide the bean mixture between two plates. When the fish is done (about 5 minutes on the second side) place the filets on top of the beans. Top the fish with the chilled tomato vinaigrette and serve.

Nutrition Facts	
Serving size	4 oz. fish with beans
Servings	4
Calories 453	Calories from Fat 119
	% Daily Value
Total Fat 14 g	21 %
Saturated Fat 2 g	12 %
Trans Fat 0 g	
Monounsaturated Fat 8 g	
Cholesterol 54 mg	18 %
Sodium 604 mg	25 %
Total Carbohydrates 49 g	16 %
Dietary Fiber 14 g	54 %
Sugars 5 g	
Protein 37 g	
Vitamin A 130 %	Vitamin C 25 %
Calcium 15 %	Iron 25 %
Vitamin K 33 mcg	
Potassium 1407 mg	
Magnesium 154 mg	

Pepperoni Pizza

1 **30 min.**

Serving size = 1 pizza

This recipe can easily be multiplied by 2, 3 or 4. Leftovers are good cold for breakfast. This recipe requires Pizza Dough and Tomato Sauce be made first (recipes included).

1/4 cup	Tomato Sauce
1/4 cup	shredded part skim milk mozzarella
1/2 oz.	Hormel Turkey Pepperoni (about 8 slices)
1/4 recipe	whole wheat pizza dough

Pizza is best baked on a pizza stone but a cookie sheet will work as well. Place the baking stone or cookie sheet in an oven that has been preheated to 500°F. Allow the baking suface to heat for at least 15-20 minutes.

Using 1/4 of the pizza dough recipe (for each pizza), gently stretch into 8-inch rounds. Don't work too hard to get a perfectly round shape.

Once the dough is formed, place it on top of the hot pizza stone and top with 1/4 cup marinara sauce. Place the pepperoni discs on top of the sauce and top with the shredded mozzarella.

Bake for approximately ten to twelve minutes until the crust is golden brown.

"Believe it or not, Americans eat 75 acres of pizza a day."

Boyd Matson, National Geographic explorer

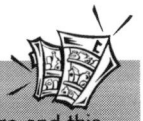

The refrigerator light goes on...
You deserve your share of that acreage and this pizza is the real deal. If you don't want to make your own tomato sauce, using one of the bottled sauces works fine. The Newman's Own® Marinara sauce is a good choice and not too terribly high in sodium (it will add about 225 mg of sodium to this recipe). It has a good sweet flavor that's just right for pizza. You can also look for a low-sodium tomato sauce if you are on a salt restricted diet – they are much easier to find these days.

Nutrition Facts	
Serving size	1 pizza (includes dough and toppings)
Servings	1
Calories 422	Calories from Fat 82
	% Daily Value
Total Fat 9 g	14 %
Saturated Fat 4 g	22 %
Trans Fat 0 g	
Monounsaturated Fat 3 g	
Cholesterol 32 mg	11 %
Sodium 702 mg	29 %
Total Carbohydrates 66 g	22 %
Dietary Fiber 9 g	35 %
Sugars 8 g	
Protein 22 g	
Vitamin A 5 %	Vitamin C 13 %
Calcium 26 %	Iron 25 %
Vitamin K 4 mcg	
Potassium 528 mg	
Magnesium 109 mg	

Pizza with Dill Pesto and Potato

1 **30 min.**

Serving size = 1 pizza

This recipe can easily be multiplied by 2, 3 or 4. This recipe doesn't keep well. This recipe requires Whole Wheat Pizza Dough and Dill Pesto to be made first (recipes included).

1 quart	water
2	small red potatoes (about 4 oz)
2 Tbsp.	dill pesto
1/2 oz.	fresh mozzarella (cut into small dice)
1/4 recipe	whole wheat pizza dough
to taste	fresh ground pepper

Place the water in a stock pot over high heat. Bring to a boil and add the potatoes. Cook the potatoes until slightly tender. Remove and allow them to cool. Slice into rounds about 1/4 inch thick

Pizza is best baked on a pizza stone but a cookie sheet will work as well. Place the baking stone or cookie sheet in an oven that has been preheated to 500°F.

Using 1/4 of the pizza dough recipe (for each pizza), and gently stretch into 8 inch rounds. Don't work too hard to get a perfectly round shape.

Once the dough is formed, place the pizza dough on a floured peel and spread the pesto over the dough. Top with slices of potato and sprinkle with the mozzarella.

Place the pizza on the heated pizza stone and bake for about 12 – 15 minutes until the crust is golden brown.

"We live in an age when pizza gets to your home before the police."

Jeff Arder, Comedian

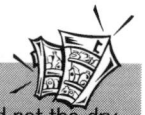

The refrigerator light goes on...
This recipe uses fresh mozzarella and not the dry, shredded American type that pizza joints use. Fresh mozzarella is so rich and melts wonderfully. You'll love it with the Dill Pesto and potatoes.

Nutrition Facts	
Serving size	1 pizza (includes dough and toppings)
Servings	2
Calories 502	Calories from Fat 116
	% Daily Value
Total Fat 13 g	21 %
Saturated Fat 4 g	18 %
Trans Fat 0 g	
Monounsaturated Fat 6 g	
Cholesterol 14 mg	5 %
Sodium 453 mg	19 %
Total Carbohydrates 82 g	27 %
Dietary Fiber 11 g	43 %
Sugars 7 g	
Protein 18 g	
Vitamin A 11 %	Vitamin C 46 %
Calcium 18 %	Iron 27 %
Vitamin K 9 mcg	
Potassium 843 mg	
Magnesium 133 mg	

Baked Penne

6 **60 min.**

Serving size = 2.67 ounces pasta

I would not multiply this recipe. This recipe is a meal unto itself and requires no side dishes. Leftovers are great! They can be divided and placed in ziplock bags and frozen.

1 large	yellow pepper
2 large	red pepper
1 lb.	eggplant (cut into 1 inch cubes)
6 small	shallots (peeled)
1 lb.	penne (whole wheat is best)
5 quarts	water
1/4 cup	egg substitute
2 Tbsp.	fresh oregano (coarsely chopped)
1 ounce	pecorino-romano (grated)
1/4 tsp.	salt
	pepper to taste
2 tsp.	unsalted butter
3 oz.	fontina cheese (shredded)

Preheat the oven to 375°F.

Seed the peppers and cut into 1 inch squares. Place the eggplant, shallots and peppers in a roasting pan and lightly spray with olive oil. Place the roasting pan in the preheated oven and roast the vegetables until slightly soft (about 15 – 20 minutes).

While the vegetables are roasting bring 5 quarts of water to a boil and add the penne. Cook until slightly underdone (about 12 – 15 minutes). Drain.

Prepare a 12" oblong pan (pyrex is a good choice) by lightly spraying the inside with olive oil. Set aside. (Lining the pan with Release non-stick foil works well also).

Place the egg substitute, oregano, Romano cheese, salt and pepper in a glass or stainless steel bowl. Stir well and add the penne and butter. Toss the pasta to coat well.
Add the vegetables and fold together gently until well blended. Pour the ingredients into the prepared oblong pan.

Sprinkle the grated fontina over the top. Bake at 375° for 15 - 20 minutes until the top is lightly browned.

"How can anyone govern a nation that has 246 different kinds of cheese?"

Charles de Gaulle,
President of France

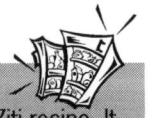

The refrigerator light goes on...
This is a creamy version of a Baked Ziti recipe. It is a similar recipe and not many more calories. It is still pretty healthy with only 19% of calories from fat, but if you are working on your weight you might eat a smaller portion.

Nutrition Facts	
Serving size	2.67 oz. pasta
Servings	6
Calories 446	Calories from Fat 79
	% Daily Value
Total Fat 9 g	14 %
Saturated Fat 5 g	24 %
Trans Fat 0 g	
Monounsaturated Fat 2 g	
Cholesterol 25 mg	8 %
Sodium 300 mg	12 %
Total Carbohydrates 74 g	25 %
Dietary Fiber 9 g	35 %
Sugars 11 g	
Protein 19 g	
Vitamin A 119 %	Vitamin C 369 %
Calcium 18 %	Iron 23 %
Vitamin K 14 mcg	
Potassium 822 mg	
Magnesium 81 mg	

Barbecue Chicken

1 **30 min.**

Serving size = 1 piece chicken

This recipe can easily be multiplied by up to eight. Leftovers are great.

1 cup	low-sodium ketchup
1/4 cup	apricot jelly
1/4 cup	dark brown sugar
1/2 cup	cider vinegar
1 Tbsp.	Worcestershire sauce
2 tsp.	water
1/8 tsp.	hot sauce
1/8 tsp.	garlic powder
1/2 tsp.	dry mustard
1 tsp.	chili powder
1 tsp.	paprika
1 tsp.	ground black pepper
1 piece per serving	chicken (breast, thigh, drumstick) (skin removed)

Mix all ingredients, except the chicken, in a blender and chill overnight.

Heat grill to medium heat (approx. 350°F).

Dip chicken pieces in barbecue sauce and place on grill. Turn frequently, spreading the rest of the sauce on the chicken as it cooks.

"Ketchup has natural mellowing agents."
The Ketchup Advisory Board, advertising on Prairie Home Companion

The refrigerator light goes on...
Barbecue sauce is a funny thing. Religion for some and with good reason. The complexities of making a good sauce are debated endlessly. This recipe relies heavily on the brown sugar and jam to create a caramelized glaze on whatever you decide to use it on.

Sugar adds calories plain and simple. If you are really watching calories there are a lot of sauces out there with fewer calories and are actually pretty low in sodium. I use them actually more often than I make my own. I look for ones that are low in both calories and sodium. One of my recent favorites is Arriba!® Fire Roasted Chipotle Bar-B-Q Sauce. Full of flavor, 1/4 cup has only 20 calories and only 300 mg sodium.

Nutrition Facts	
Serving size	1 piece chicken
Servings	8
Calories 217	Calories from Fat 15
	% Daily Value
Total Fat 2 g	3 %
Saturated Fat 0 g	2 %
Trans Fat 0 g	
Monounsaturated Fat 0 g	
Cholesterol 68 mg	23 %
Sodium 126 mg	5 %
Total Carbohydrates 21 g	7 %
Dietary Fiber 0 g	2 %
Sugars 18 g	
Protein 28 g	
Vitamin A 10 %	Vitamin C 13 %
Calcium 3 %	Iron 8 %
Vitamin K 2 mcg	
Potassium 482 mg	
Magnesium 43 mg	

Ginger Cilantro Flank Steak

4 **60 min.**

Serving size = 4 ounces beef

To multiply make separate bags of marinade with steak. Leftovers are fantastic and make good sandwiches and salads.

1 lb.	flank steak
3 Tbsp.	fresh ginger (minced)
1 Tbsp.	dark sesame oil
1 Tbsp.	low-sodium soy sauce
1 Tbsp.	rice vinegar
1 Tbsp.	Splenda
1 tsp.	hot bean paste
1/2 cup	cilantro leaves

Combine the flank steak, minced ginger, sesame oil, soy sauce, rice vinegar, Splenda, red bean paste and cilantro leaves in a zipper bag. Close the bag and toss to coat the steak well.

Marinate at least four hours in the refrigerator (overnight is best).

When you are ready to cook the steak, preheat the oven to broil or start the barbecue grill on medium-high heat.

Lightly spray a broiler or non-stick grill pan or skillet with oil. Put the flank steak on the pan and place it under the broiler (or place the steak on the grill). Cook for about 8 - 9 minutes on each side for medium-rare.

Remove to a cutting board and allow the meat to rest for about 5 to 10 minutes prior to slicing. Carve the meat as thin as possible and serve.

"Beef is the soul of cooking."
Marie-Antoine Carême,
19th century chef

The refrigerator light goes on...
Comparing this with the Garlic Lime Flank Steak shows how different a recipe can be, even though it uses the same cut of meat and the same technique—the only difference here is the marinade. This recipe is not especially spicy, but can be by simply increasing the amount of hot bean paste.

Nutrition Facts	
Serving size	4 oz. beef
Servings	4
Calories 206	Calories from Fat 95
	% Daily Value
Total Fat 11 g	16 %
Saturated Fat 3 g	17 %
Trans Fat 0 g	
Monounsaturated Fat 4 g	
Cholesterol 48 mg	16 %
Sodium 246 mg	10 %
Total Carbohydrates 1 g	0 %
Dietary Fiber 0 g	1 %
Sugars 0 g	
Protein 25 g	
Vitamin A 3 %	Vitamin C 3 %
Calcium 3 %	Iron 1 %
Vitamin K 8 mcg	
Potassium 427 mg	
Magnesium 30 mg	

Pizza with Thai Peanut Sauce and Scallops

2 **30 min.**

Serving size = 1 pizza

This recipe can easily be multiplied by 2, 3 or 4. Leftovers are good cold for breakfast. Serve with red wine (but not at breakfast) and a good movie. Make the Whole Wheat Pizza Dough and Thai Peanut Sauce first (recipes included).

1 tsp.	extra virgin olive oil
1 large	leek (cleaned & sliced into thin rounds)
2 Tbsp.	Thai Peanut Sauce
1 tsp.	extra virgin olive oil
6 - about 6 oz.	sea scallops
2 Tbsp.	unsalted dry roasted peanuts (chopped fine)
1/2 cup	fresh cilantro leaves
1/2 cup	fresh mung bean sprouts
1/2 recipe (1/4 for each pizza)	whole wheat pizza dough

Pizza is best baked on a pizza stone but a cookie sheet will work as well. Place the baking stone or cookie sheet in an oven that has been preheated to 500°F. Allow the baking surface to heat for at least 15-20 minutes.

Place 1 tsp. olive oil in a non-stick skillet pan over medium high heat. Add the leek and reduce the heat to medium. Cook until the leeks begin to soften and brown stirring frequently. Add the peanut sauce and toss to coat thoroughly. Set aside.

While the leeks are cooking, heat the remaining 1 tsp. olive oil in a small non-stick skillet over high heat. When the pan is very hot, add the scallops to the pan. Sear on one side about 3 minutes and turn. Cook on the other side for about another three minutes. Remove to a paper towel to drain.
When they are cool slice them in half so there are two discs for each scallop (a total of 6 discs per pizza)

Using 1/4 of the pizza dough recipe (for each pizza), gently stretch into 8-inch rounds. Don't work too hard to get a perfectly round shape.

Once the dough is formed, place it on top of the hot pizza stone and top each with one half of the leek mixture. Sprinkle 1-tablespoon of peanuts per pizza and top with 6 scallop discs (seared side up) and then 1/4 cup cilantro leaves per pizza.

Bake for about 10 - 12 minutes until the dough begins to brown. Top with 1/4 cup bean sprouts and cook for another 2 minutes.

"Most seafoods... should be simply threatened with heat and then celebrated with joy."
Jeff Smith, The Frugal Gourmet

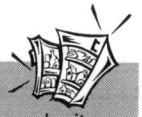

The refrigerator light goes on...
I love this recipe and you don't have to make it with the Thai Peanut Sauce recipe. There are a number of good sauces on the market and they are not too high in calories, fat or sodium. I will often substitute the Whole Foods brand when I make this pizza and it still comes in at about the same nutrition content.

Nutrition Facts	
Serving size	1 pizza (including dough)
Servings	2
Calories 465	Calories from Fat 71
	% Daily Value
Total Fat 9 g	13 %
Saturated Fat 2 g	7 %
Trans Fat 0 g	
Monounsaturated Fat 3 g	
Cholesterol 28 mg	9 %
Sodium 480 mg	20 %
Total Carbohydrates 74 g	25 %
Dietary Fiber 10 g	40 %
Sugars 9 g	
Protein 29 g	
Vitamin A 21 %	Vitamin C 18 %
Calcium 8 %	Iron 28 %
Vitamin K 39 mcg	
Potassium 768 mg	
Magnesium 173 mg	

Grilled Sage Lamb Kabob

2 **30 min.**

Serving Size = 1 kabob

This recipe can easily be multiplied by any amount. The marinade keeps well overnight.

2 Tbsp.	fresh sage
2 Tbsp.	fresh chives
1 Tbsp.	fresh lemon juice
1 Tbsp.	pure maple syrup
2 Tbsp.	dry sherry
1 Tbsp.	extra virgin olive oil
1 Tbsp.	dark brown sugar
1/4 tsp.	salt
8 oz.	lean lamb shoulder
2 cups	water
4 medium	red potatoes
1/2	medium white onion (peeled and halved)
1/2	red bell pepper
6	shiitake mushroom caps

Place the sage, chives, lemon juice, pure maple syrup, sherry, olive oil, brown sugar and salt in a blender and puree until smooth.

Cut the lamb into eight, one-ounce cubes. Combine the marinade and lamb in a zipper bag. Allow to marinate in the refrigerator at least four hours (overnight is best).

Place the water in a stock pot fitted with a steamer basket over high heat.

Cut the potatoes in half. Place the potatoes and the half onion in a steamer and steam for 15 minutes. Allow to cool.

Quarter the half onion and the pepper.

On a skewer, alternate: mushroom cap, lamb cube, quartered onion, quartered pepper and potato. Keep the marinade in reserve.

Cook kabobs over a hot grill. Turn about every three minutes and baste with the remaining marinade as the kabobs cook.

"My kids always perceived the bathroom as a place where you wait it out until all the groceries are unloaded from the car."

Erma Bombeck, Iconic housewife

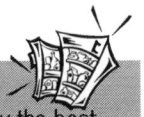

The refrigerator light goes on...
More proof that red meat is okay. Buy the best quality New Zealand lamb and trim it well. Pair it with good aromatic herbs, such as sage or rosemary, and you can't go wrong.

Nutrition Facts	
Serving size	1 lamb kabob
Servings	2
Calories 627	Calories from Fat 126
	% Daily Value
Total Fat 14 g	22 %
Saturated Fat 4 g	19 %
Trans Fat 0 g	
Monounsaturated Fat 8 g	
Cholesterol 69 mg	23 %
Sodium 420 mg	17 %
Total Carbohydrates 92 g	31 %
Dietary Fiber 9 g	36 %
Sugars 22 g	
Protein 33 g	
Vitamin A 80 %	Vitamin C 279 %
Calcium 5 %	Iron 25 %
Vitamin K 33 mcg	
Potassium 2741 mg	
Magnesium 137 mg	

Gnocchi

2 **45 min.**

Serving size = 10 gnocchi

This recipe can be multiplied by 2. Leftovers are fair at best. I have kept the gnocchi refrigerated overnight but they are not as good as when fresh. Serve with Dill Pesto or Tomato Sauce (recipes included). Nutrition information is for the gnocchi only.

10 oz.	yukon gold potatoes
6 Tbsp.	all purpose white flour
1 large	egg
1/4 tsp.	salt
1/8 tsp.	ground nutmeg
1/8 tsp.	ground black pepper
4 quarts	water

Peel the potatoes, rinse and cut into 1-inch cubes. Place a steamer basket in a large sauce pan. Add about 1 1/2 cups water and set the pan over high heat. Steam the cubed potatoes until very tender (about 20 minutes). Remove the steamer basket and allow the potatoes to cool until they are no more than warm to the touch.

Force all of the steamed potatoes through a potato ricer into a large mixing bowl. (If you don't have a potato ricer, the potatoes must be chopped until there are no lumps. Do not over mash them or the gnocchi will be pasty.)

Add 3 tablespoons of the flour to the potatoes with the egg, salt, nutmeg and black pepper. Mix together using a fork. The mixture will take on a crumbly consistency. Add 2 tablespoons of the remaining flour and blend well.

Knead the dough gently until all the flour is blended in. Stop kneading when the flour is incorporated. After the dough is smooth, cut it into 2 equal pieces. Place one tablespoon of flour on a cutting board and roll each piece of dough into a rope about as big around as your thumb. Cut the ropes in 1/2 inch pieces (about ten per roll) and then roll the dumpling over the tines of a fork to shape the ridges of the gnocchi.
Boil at least 4 quarts of water and add the gnocchi no more than 2 servings at a time (20 gnocchi). As they float to the top of the water, they are done. Remove them and add to prepared sauce.

"I think they should just throw a bag of gnocchi up in the air; it would fill up the hole."
Jennifer Boyer

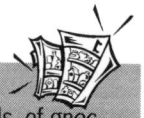

The refrigerator light goes on...
There are hundreds, maybe thousands, of gnocchi recipes. Most of the basic recipes, much like pasta, are mostly carbohydrates and are low in fat. There are recipes that contain all different ingredients – from mushrooms to cheese to pesto. Choose the ingredients that might add more calories carefully, but do choose them. Making gnocchi is great fun and, with a bit of practice, you can create light fluffy pillows to swim in your sauces.

Nutrition Facts	
Serving size	10 gnocchi
Servings	8
Calories 239	Calories from Fat 26
	% Daily Value
Total Fat 3 g	4 %
Saturated Fat 1 g	4 %
Trans Fat 0 g	
Monounsaturated Fat 1 g	
Cholesterol 106 mg	35 %
Sodium 322 mg	13 %
Total Carbohydrates 45 g	15 %
Dietary Fiber 3 g	13 %
Sugars 1 g	
Protein 8 g	
Vitamin A 3 %	Vitamin C 17 %
Calcium 3 %	Iron 11 %
Vitamin K 3 mcg	
Potassium 517 mg	
Magnesium 36 mg	

Tomato Sauce

Servings = 10
Serving size = 1/2 cup
Makes 5 cups

Keeps well in the fridge for about 4 – 5 days.

1 Tbsp.	olive oil
6 cloves	garlic (minced)
1	small onion (diced)
2 – 28 oz. cans	no salt added peeled tomatoes (chopped)
3 cups	water
1/4 tsp	salt

Place the oil in a large skillet and heat over a medium-high heat. Reduce the heat to medium and add the garlic. Cook gently for about 3 minutes. Do not allow the garlic to turn brown.

Add the onions and cook until they are translucent. Stir frequently and do not allow them to brown.

Add the tomatoes and water and reduce the heat to low. Cook until the tomatoes are soft (about 90 minutes).

Remove from heat, add the salt and puree until smooth with a stick or conventional blender.

There is no love sincerer than the love of food.
George Bernard Shaw, Playwright

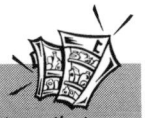

The refrigerator light goes on...
This recipe is based on a can of tomatoes that has about 425 mg of sodium per serving.

Nutrition Facts	
Serving size	1/2 cup
Servings	10
Calories 43	Calories from Fat 14
	% Daily Value
Total Fat 2 g	2 %
Saturated Fat 0 g	1 %
Trans Fat 0 g	
Monounsaturated Fat 0 g	
Cholesterol 0 mg	0 %
Sodium 21 mg	1 %
Total Carbohydrates 7 g	2 %
Dietary Fiber 2 g	7 %
Sugars 4 g	
Protein 1 g	
Vitamin A 4 %	Vitamin C 26 %
Calcium 5 %	Iron 9 %
Vitamin K 5 mcg	
Potassium 311 mg	
Magnesium 18 mg	

Mustard Seared Whitefish

2 **30 min.**

Serving size = 4 ounces fish

This recipe can easily be multiplied by 2, 3, 4, 5, 6.
This recipe does not make very good leftovers.

1 large	egg
3 tsp.	olive oil
2 tsp.	Dijon mustard
1/8 tsp.	salt
1/8 tsp.	paprika
1 Tbsp.	dried sage (crumbled)
to taste	fresh ground black pepper
2 - 4 oz.	whitefish filets (trout, cod, drum, tilapia)

Whisk together the egg, 1 teaspoon of the olive oil, Dijon mustard, salt, paprika, sage and black pepper until smooth. Put the mixture in the refrigerator.

Place a large skillet in the oven and preheat to 400°F.

While the oven is preheating rinse the fish filets and pat dry with a paper towel.

When the oven is hot add the remaining 2 teaspoons of olive oil to the pan. Dredge both sides of the fish in the mustard coating and place them in the hot pan.

Return the pan to the oven and cook for about 4 minutes on the first side. Turn the fish over. Change the setting of the oven to broil and cook for about another 3 - 4 minutes. Serve.

"What is special about Fisher is not the tedious stuff about six teaspoons of dry mustard, but the literary dressing around the sides of the recipes."
Philip Howard, Author

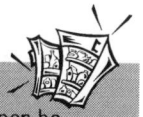

The refrigerator light goes on...
The one key to this recipe is that the pan be very hot because the egg wash sears onto the fish when it hits the pan. Timing is everything in making the perfect fish recipe. Have the fish ready and already coated on one side. Remove the pan from the oven, add the oil, and swirl it around the pan. Coat the other side of the filets and add them to the pan quickly.

Nutrition Facts	
Serving size	4 oz. fish
Servings	2
Calories 265	Calories from Fat 151
	% Daily Value
Total Fat 1 g	26 %
Saturated Fat 3 g	15 %
Trans Fat 0 g	
Monounsaturated Fat 10 g	
Cholesterol 171 mg	57 %
Sodium 301 mg	13 %
Total Carbohydrates 1 g	0 %
Dietary Fiber 0 g	1 %
Sugars 0 g	
Protein 27 g	
Vitamin A 5 %	Vitamin C 1 %
Calcium 6 %	Iron 13 %
Vitamin K 4 mcg	
Potassium 448 mg	
Magnesium 30 mg	

Pan-Seared Pork Chops with Savory Peach Marmalade

4 **45 min.**

Serving size = 4 ounces pork with sauce.

This recipe can easily be multiplied by 2 or halved. This recipe makes good leftovers. Serve with Mashed Yams (recipe included).

2 Tbsp	olive oil
1	clove garlic (peeled and sliced)
2 tsp	dry rubbed sage
1 small	Vidalia (or sweet) onion (diced)
1 pound	peaches, peeled & sliced thinly
1/2 cup	non-fat chicken stock
1/4 cup	water
1	lime, juiced
1/2 tsp	salt
1/4 tsp	ground cumin
to taste	fresh ground black pepper
2 tsp..	maple syrup
2 tsp.	unsalted butter
4 4-oz.	center cut pork chops, boneless
1/4	red bell pepper, finely diced

Place a medium stainless steel or non-reactive saucepan over medium heat. Add 1 Tbsp. olive oil, garlic, and sage, cook for one minute, stirring frequently.

Add diced onion and cook for three minutes. Add sliced peaches and 1/2 cup chicken stock. Reduce heat to low. Add water, lime juice, 1/4 tsp. salt, ground cumin, and black pepper, and stir well. Cook, simmering gently, for 20 minutes, until peaches are softened.

Gently mash peaches with a fork until they're the consistency of marmalade. Add 2 tsps butter and set aside. Place a large skillet in oven and preheat oven to 375F.

When hot, sprinkle the remaining 1/4 tsp salt over the pork chops. Add the remaining 1 tbsp olive oil to the hot pan. Place the pork chops in the pan, seasoned side down.
Put back in the oven and cook for 7-9 minutes, then turn. Cook for an additional 5-6 minutes. Plate each pork chop and serve, topped with the peach marmalade and sprinkled with 1/4 diced red pepper.

"Life is better than death, I believe, if only because it is less boring and because it has fresh peaches in it."

Thomas Walker, Physician

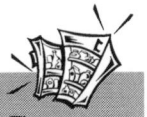

The refrigerator light goes on...
I love the flavor of peaches with pork. They seem so right together. The addition of the sage and onions makes this simple topping for pork just a bit savory. This is a good example of using fats that are good for you like the olive oil with just a little butter to enhance the flavor and texture of the cooked peaches. It doesn't take much – just a bit to finish off the sauce.

Nutrition Facts	
Serving size	4 oz. pork with sauce
Servings	4
Calories 309	Calories from Fat 146
	% Daily Value
Total Fat 16 g	25 %
Saturated Fat 5 g	24 %
Trans Fat 0 g	
Monounsaturated Fat 9 g	
Cholesterol 67 mg	22 %
Sodium 354 mg	15 %
Total Carbohydrates 14 g	5 %
Dietary Fiber 2 g	7 %
Sugars 9 g	
Protein 27 g	
Vitamin A 11 %	Vitamin C 40 %
Calcium 3 %	Iron 7 %
Vitamin K 9 mcg	
Potassium 721 mg	
Magnesium 38 mg	

Turkey Burgers

2 **30 min.**

Serving size = 1 - 1/4 lb. burger.

This recipe can easily be multiplied by 2, 3, 4. This recipe does not make very good leftovers.

8 ounces	ground turkey (breast is better)
1/4 tsp.	salt
to taste	fresh ground black pepper
1 tsp.	extra virgin olive oil
1/4 tsp.	dried thyme leaves
2 - 3/4 oz. slices	reduced fat Swiss cheese
2	whole wheat hamburger buns
	lettuce
	tomato
	onions

Place a non-stick grill pan in the oven. Preheat to 375°F.

Combine the turkey, salt, pepper, olive oil and thyme leaves until well blended. Divide into two balls and form into a burger.

When the oven is hot place the burgers in the grill pan. Cook on the first side for about ten minutes.

After turning cook for about 5 - 7 minutes and top with the cheese. Cook until the cheese is melted.

Serve with 1 tablespoon non-fat mayonnaise, lettuce, tomato and onions.

"Rock and roll is the hamburger that ate the world."

Peter York, Musician

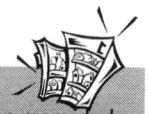

The refrigerator light goes on...
Most ground turkey is mixed and often more dark meat than breast meat. Ask your butcher for breast meat if it's available. There's a lot less fat and the burgers will be a little more tender. If you do use breast meat only, there's more need for the oil or the burgers will be dry.

If you can only get dark meat, you will find less need for the oil.

Nutrition Facts	
Serving size	1 burger
Servings	4
Calories 343	Calories from Fat 58
	% Daily Value
Total Fat 6 g	10 %
Saturated Fat 2 g	9 %
Trans Fat 0 g	
Monounsaturated Fat 3 g	
Cholesterol 78 mg	26 %
Sodium787 mg	33 %
Total Carbohydrates 28 g	9 %
Dietary Fiber 5 g	19 %
Sugars 6 g	
Protein 41 g	
Vitamin A 13 %	Vitamin C 10 %
Calcium 28 %	Iron 16 %
Vitamin K 39 mcg	
Potassium 600 mg	
Magnesium 90 mg	

Cocktail Sauce

Servings = 4
Serving size = about 4 tablespoons.

This recipe can easily be multiplied by 2 or 3.
This keeps well for about a week in the fridge.

3/4 cup	no salt added ketchup
3 Tbsp.	prepared horseradish
2 Tbsp.	fresh lemon juice
1/4 tsp.	hot sauce
1/ tsp.	salt
to taste	fresh ground black pepper

Mix all ingredients together until well blended. Chill for at least an hour before serving.

"You can't have everything. Where would you put it?"

Steven Wright, Comic

The refrigerator light goes on...
This is a good example of using a low-sodium food and then adding a measured amount of salt to the recipe for flavor but still being able to control the total amount.

Nutrition Facts	
Serving size	1/4 cup
Servings	4
Calories 55	Calories from Fat 0
	% Daily Value
Total Fat 0 g	0 %
Saturated Fat 0 g	0 %
Trans Fat 0 g	
Monounsaturated Fat 0 g	
Cholesterol 0 mg	0 %
Sodium 191 mg	8 %
Total Carbohydrates 13 g	5 %
Dietary Fiber 1 g	2 %
Sugars 11 g	
Protein 1 g	
Vitamin A 9 %	Vitamin C 22 %
Calcium 2 %	Iron 2 %
Vitamin K 1 mcg	
Potassium 209 mg	
Magnesium 12 mg	

Thai Peanut Sauce

Servings = 8
Serving size = 2 tablespoons peanut sauce

This recipe can easily be multiplied by 2, 3 or 4. This sauce will keep for about 3 weeks sealed tightly in the refrigerator.

1/4 cup	reduced-fat peanut butter
6 Tbsp.	chicken stock
1/4 cup	reduced-fat (lite) unsweetened coconut milk
2 tsp.	low-sodium soy sauce
2 tsp.	rice vinegar
2 tsp.	Tabasco sauce

Combine the reduced-fat peanut butter, chicken stock, reduced-fat coconut milk, low-sodium soy sauce, rice vinegar and Tabasco in a small bowl. Whisk until smooth and set aside. (This can be made up to 48 hours in advance and refrigerated).

"I eat at this German-Chinese restaurant and the food is delicious. The only problem is that an hour later you're hungry for power."

Dick Cavett, Television personality

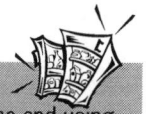

The refrigerator light goes on...
Peanut sauce is a staple of Thai cuisine and using the lower calorie and lower fat ingredients makes this possible. These are ingredients that I always have in my pantry and you should too.

Nutrition Facts	
Serving size	2 Tbsp. sauce
Servings	8
Calories 45	Calories from Fat 25
	% Daily Value
Total Fat 3 g	4 %
Saturated Fat 1 g	4 %
Trans Fat 0 g	
Monounsaturated Fat 0 g	
Cholesterol 0 mg	0 %
Sodium 93 mg	6 %
Total Carbohydrates 3 g	1 %
Dietary Fiber 0 g	2 %
Sugars 1 g	
Protein 2 g	
Vitamin A 0 %	Vitamin C 0 %
Calcium 0 %	Iron 1 %
Vitamin K 0 mcg	
Potassium 61 mg	
Magnesium 13 mg	

Roasted Garlic

Servings = 6
Serving size =1/3 head of garlic (about 4-6 cloves)

I make up to about 4 heads of garlic at a time. This keeps well, tightly covered, for about 4 - 6 days.

2	heads whole garlic
2 tsps.	extra virgin olive oil

Preheat oven to 300°F.

Peel the outermost skin of the garlic only. With the bulb whole, turn on its side and slice 1/2-inch of the stem end off the garlic bulbs.

Pour the olive oil in the bottom of a heavy bottom sauce pan.

Place the garlic cut side down in the pan.

Cover and roast for 45 minutes until cloves are slightly brown at the cut end and soft throughout.

"There is no such thing as a little garlic."
Arthur Baer, Investment Author

The refrigerator light goes on...
Roasted garlic is a staple in my kitchen and should be in yours. I generally roast about 3 heads every ten days or so. It makes a great ingredient in mashed potatoes and also enriches any sauce. It is fantastic served as hors d'oeuvres on bread with some soft goat cheese and veggies.

Nutrition Facts	
Serving size	1/3 head of garlic (about 4-6 cloves)
Servings	6
Calories 40	Calories from Fat 14
	% Daily Value
Total Fat 2 g	2 %
Saturated Fat 0 g	1 %
Trans Fat 0 g	
Monounsaturated Fat 0 g	
Cholesterol 0 mg	0 %
Sodium 3 mg	0 %
Total Carbohydrates 6 g	2 %
Dietary Fiber 0 g	2 %
Sugars 0 g	
Protein 1 g	
Vitamin A 0 %	Vitamin C 9 %
Calcium 3 %	Iron 2 %
Vitamin K 1 mcg	
Potassium 72 mg	
Magnesium 5 mg	

Candied Carrots

Servings = 2
Serving size = about one cup carrots

This recipe can easily be multiplied by 2 or 3. This recipe does not make very good leftovers.

2 cups	water
8 oz.	carrots (peeled and sliced)
1 Tbsp.	light spread
1 Tbsp.	maple syrup
1/4 tsp.	salt

Place the water in a pot fitted with a steamer basket over high heat.Steam for about 10 -15 minutes until the carrots are slightly tender.

Combine the cooked carrots with the light spread, maple syrup and salt and serve.

"An intellectual carrot. The mind boggles."
Lederer and Nyby, Screenwriters
of The Thing from Another World

The refrigerator light goes on...
Most candied carrots recipes are way too sweet and the amount of brown sugar or molasses or maple syrup masks the flavor of the carrots. The combination of the light spread and a small amount of maple syrup with the salt balances nicely with the natural sweetness of the carrots.

Nutrition Facts	
Serving size	1 cup
Servings	4
Calories 96	Calories from Fat 26
	% Daily Value
Total Fat 3 g	4 %
Saturated Fat 1 g	4 %
Trans Fat 0 g	
Monounsaturated Fat 1 g	
Cholesterol 0 mg	0 %
Sodium 276 mg	11 %
Total Carbohydrates 18 g	6 %
Dietary Fiber 3 g	13 %
Sugars 11 g	
Protein 1 g	
Vitamin A 391 %	Vitamin C 11 %
Calcium 4 %	Iron 3 %
Vitamin K 17 mcg	
Potassium 387 mg	
Magnesium 15 mg	

Coconut Rice

Servings = 2
Serving size = 1/2 cup rice

This recipe can easily be multiplied by 2, 3 or 4.
The cooked rice doesn't keep well.

1/2 cup	reduced-fat (lite) unsweetened coconut milk
3/4 cup	water
1/4 tsp.	salt
1/2 cup	jasmine rice

Prior to opening the can of coconut milk, shake very well.

In a medium sauce pain, heat the coconut milk, water and salt. When the liquid boils, stir in the jasmine rice.

Reduce heat to medium-low and simmer, covered, for about 15 minutes.

Do not boil away all of the liquid and do not stir the rice.

When a very small amount of liquid remains, remove the pan from the burner and let it stand, covered, for 5 minutes before serving.

"Rice is a beautiful food. It is beautiful when it grows, precision rows of sparkling green stalks shooting up to reach the hot summer sun. It is beautiful when harvested, autumn gold sheaves piled on diked, patchwork paddies. It is beautiful when, once threshed, it enters granary bins like a (flood) of tiny seed-pearls. It is beautiful when cooked by a practiced hand, pure white and sweetly fragrant."

Shizuo Tsuji, Japanese chef
and cookbook author

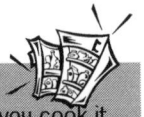

The refrigerator light goes on...
Never stir rice. It doesn't matter how you cook it, stirring it breaks down the starches on the outer layer and turns the rice to a gooey paste. Simply place the rice in the boiling liquid, stir once and cover. Leave it alone until the water is evaporated.

Nutrition Facts	
Serving size	1/2 cup rice
Servings	2
Calories 211	Calories from Fat 35
	% Daily Value
Total Fat 4 g	6 %
Saturated Fat 3 g	14 %
Trans Fat 0 g	
Monounsaturated Fat 0 g	
Cholesterol 0 mg	0 %
Sodium 304 mg	13 %
Total Carbohydrates 38 g	13 %
Dietary Fiber 1 g	2 %
Sugars 1 g	
Protein 3 g	
Vitamin A 0 %	Vitamin C 0 %
Calcium 2 %	Iron 12 %
Vitamin K 0 mcg	
Potassium 53 mg	
Magnesium 12 mg	

Jasmine Rice

Servings = 2
Serving size = 1/2 cup rice

This recipe can easily be multiplied by 2, 3 or 4.
The rice doesn't keep well.

1 cup	water
1/4 tsp.	salt
1/2 cup	jasmine rice

In a medium sauce pan, heat the water and salt. When the water boils, stir in the jasmine rice.

Reduce heat to medium-low and simmer, partially covered, for about 15 minutes.

Do not boil away all of the liquid and do not stir the rice.

When a very small amount of liquid remains, remove the pan from the burner and let it stand, covered, for 5 minutes before serving.

"Rice is the best, the most nutritive and unquestionably the most widespread staple in the world."

Auguste Escoffier, 19th century French chef

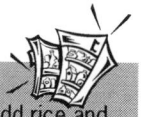

The refrigerator light goes on...
Simple, simple, simple... When you add rice and salt to water and simmer and you don't stir the result is perfect.

Nutrition Facts	
Serving size	about 1/2 cup cooked rice
Servings	2
Calories 169	Calories from Fat 0
	% Daily Value
Total Fat 0 g	0 %
Saturated Fat 0 g	0 %
Trans Fat 0 g	
Monounsaturated Fat 0 g	
Cholesterol 0 mg	0 %
Sodium 293 mg	12 %
Total Carbohydrates 37 g	12 %
Dietary Fiber <1 g	2 %
Sugars 0 g	
Protein 3 g	
Vitamin A 0 %	Vitamin C 0 %
Calcium 1 %	Iron 11 %
Vitamin K 0 mcg	
Potassium 53 mg	
Magnesium 13 mg	

Herbed Zucchini

Servings = 4
Serving size = about 2/3 cup

This recipe can easily be multiplied by 2 using a large skillet. This recipe does not make very good leftovers.

1 Tbsp.	olive oil
1 lb.	zucchini (cut into 1/4 inch dice)
2 Tbsp.	fresh herbs of your choice (minced)
1/4 tsp.	salt
to taste	fresh ground black pepper

Place the olive oil in a large non-stick skillet over medium-high heat. When the oil is hot add the zucchini. Let the zucchini cook without stirring for about 3 minutes. If it appears to be cooking too fast, reduce the heat to medium.

Toss the zucchini well and cook for about 7 - 10 more minutes. As the cubes begin to brown add the herbs, salt and pepper and continue to toss.

Do not over cook the zucchini. As soon as the outside is lightly browned and it is slightly soft, serve.

"If one consults enough herbals... every sickness known to humanity will be listed as being cured by sage."

Varro Taylor, Ph.D.,
Pharmacologist

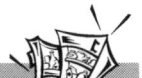

The refrigerator light goes on...
The choice of herbs here is not important. Use what you have in the garden or the fridge. Equal amounts of basil, chive, sage, rosemary and oregano will do but you could just as easily choose thyme, sage, marjoram and tarragon. This recipe will work with dried herbs but it just isn't quite as good somehow.

Nutrition Facts	
Serving size	about 2/3 cup
Servings	4
Calories 51	Calories from Fat 32
	% Daily Value
Total Fat 4 g	6 %
Saturated Fat 1 g	3 %
Trans Fat 0 g	
Monounsaturated Fat 3 g	
Cholesterol 0 mg	0 %
Sodium 88 mg	4 %
Total Carbohydrates 5 g	2 %
Dietary Fiber 2 g	7 %
Sugars 2 g	
Protein 2 g	
Vitamin A 6 %	Vitamin C 33 %
Calcium 4 %	Iron 8 %
Vitamin K 26 mcg	
Potassium 321 mg	
Magnesium 23 mg	

Green Beans with Walnut Vinaigrette

Servings = 6
Serving size = 4 ounces green beans

This recipe can easily be multiplied by 2. This recipe keeps well but the beans will turn gray-green in the refrigerator.

2 Tbsp.	shallot (minced)
2 Tbsp.	fresh lemon juice
1/4 cup	red wine vinegar
2 Tbsp.	extra virgin olive oil
1 oz.	pure walnut extract
1/4 tsp.	salt
1 tsp.	granulated sugar
2 cups	water
1-1/2 lb.	fresh green beans (trimmed at ends)

Combine the shallot, lemon juice, vinegar, walnut extract and salt in a mixing bowl.

Slowly add the oil while whisking to blend completely.

Add the sugar 1/4 tsp. at a time to adjust for acidity to taste.

Chill completely in freezer whisking occasionally so the dressing doesn't freeze.

Place the water in a medium stock pot and set a steamer basket inside the pot. Place the pot on the range over high heat. Steam the green beans until they turn bright green and are slightly tender. This will take 10 - 15 minutes. Toss the beans at about five minutes and again at ten minutes so they cook evenly.

Remove them from the heat and place in the cold vinaigrette immediately. Toss for about 2 minutes until coated well. Chill.

Serve as soon as chilled (this can be kept for days but the beans will slowly turn gray green and not look as fresh).

"Vinegar, the son of wine."
Italian Proverb

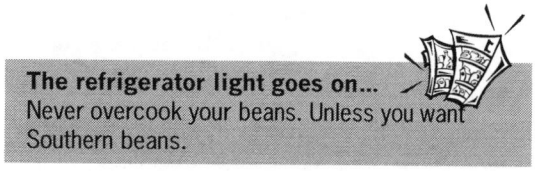

The refrigerator light goes on...
Never overcook your beans. Unless you want Southern beans.

Nutrition Facts	
Serving size	4 oz. green beans
Servings	6
Calories 96	Calories from Fat 41
	% Daily Value
Total Fat 5 g	7 %
Saturated Fat 1 g	3 %
Trans Fat 0 g	
Monounsaturated Fat 3 g	
Cholesterol 0 mg	0 %
Sodium 105 mg	4 %
Total Carbohydrates 10 g	3 %
Dietary Fiber 4 g	15 %
Sugars 3 g	
Protein 2 g	
Vitamin A 16 %	Vitamin C 35 %
Calcium 4 %	Iron 7 %
Vitamin K 19 mcg	
Potassium 262 mg	
Magnesium 30 mg	

Roasted Garlic Mashed Potatoes

Servings = 4
Serving size = about one cup.

This recipe can easily halved or be multiplied by 2 or 3. These do not keep very well. This recipe requires Roasted Garlic (recipe included) to be made first.

3 quarts	water
1 lb.	yukon gold potatoes
2 tsp.	unsalted butter
1/3 cup	non-fat buttermilk
1/3 cup	2 % milk
1/2 tsp.	salt
4 cloves	roasted garlic

Place the water in a large stockpot over high heat.

Quarter the potatoes and add them to the stock-pot. Cover with water by about an inch. Bring to boil and then reduce heat until the water is simmering.

Cook the potatoes about 15 – 20 minutes, until slightly soft in the middle. They should give when squeezed.

Remove from heat and drain water. Add butter, buttermilk, milk, salt and roasted garlic. Mash potatoes until creamy and the roasted garlic is well blended. I like to leave some chunks of potatoes. If you like them smooth, be careful because over mashing will result in pasty potatoes.

Add ground black pepper to taste.

"I have made a lot of mistakes falling in love, and regretted most of them, but never the potatoes that went with them."

Nora Ephron, Screenwriter

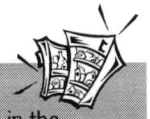

The refrigerator light goes on...
The key to good mashed potatoes is in the buttermilk / milk combination. The buttermilk adds richness and tartness, with no fat, and the milk adds creaminess. The butter is used here only as a flavor enhancer.

Nutrition Facts	
Serving size	1 cup
Servings	4
Calories 130	Calories from Fat 24
	% Daily Value
Total Fat 3 g	4 %
Saturated Fat 2 g	6 %
Trans Fat 0 g	
Monounsaturated Fat 1 g	
Cholesterol 7 mg	2 %
Sodium 176 mg	7 %
Total Carbohydrates 23 g	8 %
Dietary Fiber 3 g	10 %
Sugars 3 g	
Protein 2 g	
Vitamin A 4 %	Vitamin C 40 %
Calcium 7 %	Iron 5 %
Vitamin K 3 mcg	
Potassium 564 mg	
Magnesium 33 mg	

Green Beans with Red Onions

Servings = 4
Serving size = 4 ounces green beans

This recipe can easily be multiplied by 2. These keep well for about 48 hours in the fridge and is good served cold at picnics.

1 quart	water
1 lb.	green beans (trim the ends)
2 Tbsp.	light spread (like Promise Buttery Spread Light)
1/4 cup	red onion (diced)
1/4 tsp.	salt
1 tsp.	fresh thyme leaves
to taste	fresh ground black pepper

Place the water in a large stock pot over high heat. When the water is at a slow boil reduce the heat until the water shivers. Add the green beans and blanch for about 7 - 10 minutes until al denté.

While the beans are cooking place a large skillet over medium heat. Add the spread and as it melts toss in the red onion. Cook slowly and reduce the heat if the onion is turning brown. Stir frequently.

When the beans are done remove them from the blanching water and shake off the excess water. Add them to the red onions with the salt, thyme and black pepper.

Cook over medium heat for about two minutes and serve.

"Most people call the 'accompaniments'; just as a hat, handbag, or briefcase is to the suit, so vegetables are to the main dish."

Graham Kerr, Genius

The refrigerator light goes on...
Beans are so delicious and so good for you. These green beans will work with many different herbs. I like the taste of the thyme, however. Rosemary is wonderful as is a touch of jasmine. If you don't have the red onion, shallot will work. (White onions are fine but I like the touch of color.)

Nutrition Facts	
Serving size	4 oz. green beans
Servings	4
Calories 64	Calories from Fat 25
	% Daily Value
Total Fat 3 g	4 %
Saturated Fat 1 g	4 %
Trans Fat 0 g	
Monounsaturated Fat 1 g	
Cholesterol 0 mg	0 %
Sodium 128 mg	5 %
Total Carbohydrates 9 g	3 %
Dietary Fiber 4 g	16 %
Sugars 2 g	
Protein 2 g	
Vitamin A 23 %	Vitamin C 32 %
Calcium 5 %	Iron 8 %
Vitamin K 23 mcg	
Potassium 257 mg	
Magnesium 30 mg	

French Fries

Servings = 4
Serving size = about 4 ounces fries

This recipe can easily be multiplied by 2, but must be cooked in two batches. These do not keep very well at all.

1 lb.	russet potatoes (peeled and cut into 1/4 inch strips)
1 quart	chilled water
1 tray	ice cubes
1/2 tsp.	salt
	spray canola oil

After the potatoes are peeled and sliced, place them in a mixing bowl with cold water and ice cubes. Soak for 30 minutes.

Preheat oven to 400°F.

After soaking the potatoes, drain them and then pat dry with a paper towel.

Place the potatoes and salt in a zipper bag. Spray the potatoes for about three seconds with the canola oil and seal the zipper bag. Shake to coat the potatoes well with the oil and salt.

Carefully place the potatoes on a non-stick cookie sheet. Avoid the fries touching each other. Spray lightly with the canola oil.

Place the cookie sheet in the oven and allow the potatoes to bake for about 7 minutes. Turn the potatoes at least twice, cooking for about 7 minutes after each turn. Total cooking time will be 20 – 25 minutes.

Serve immediately.

"Zen. . . does not confuse spirituality with thinking about God while one is peeling potatoes. Zen spirituality is just to peel the potatoes."
Alan W. Watts, The Way of Zen

The refrigerator light goes on...
Oven fried foods are just like deep-fried ones, if you handle them right. Most of the time, you have to eat the dish right away. These French Fries, for instance, will keep for all of about 20 minutes (about the same amount of time as ones that have been deep fried).

Nutrition Facts	
Serving size	1/4 recipe
Servings	4
Calories 86	Calories from Fat 1
	% Daily Value
Total Fat 0 g	0 %
Saturated Fat0 g	0 %
Trans Fat 0 g	
Monounsaturated Fat 0 g	
Cholesterol 0 mg	0 %
Sodium 297 mg	12 %
Total Carbohydrates 20 g	7 %
Dietary Fiber 2 g	10 %
Sugars 1 g	
Protein 2 g	
Vitamin A 0 %	Vitamin C 37 %
Calcium 1 %	Iron 5 %
Vitamin K 2 mcg	
Potassium 472 mg	
Magnesium 26 mg	

Roasted Beets

Servings = 4
Serving size = about 1 cup beets

This recipe can easily be multiplied by 2, 3 or 4 but a larger roasting pan must be used. Leftovers are great ingredients in tossed salads.

2	medium beets
1 tsp.	unsalted butter
1/4 tsp.	salt
1/8 tsp.	dried oregano
1/8 tsp.	chili powder

Preheat the oven to 400°F.

Wrap beets in a paper towel and cook on high in microwave for 5 minutes. Let cool for 5 minutes.

Peel and cut into 1 inch cubes.

Place in a roasting pan large enough so that the beets are not completely touching.

Put the pat of butter on the beets and sprinkle the salt, oregano and chili powder over the top.

Reduce the heat to 375°F and roast for 20 – 25 minutes. The beets are done when they are slightly crisp on the outside.

"The beet is the most intense of vegetables. The radish, admittedly, is more feverish, but the fire of the radish is a cold fire, the fire of discontent, not of passion. Tomatoes are lusty enough, yet there runs through tomatoes an undercurrent of frivolity. Beets are deadly serious."

Tom Robbins, Author

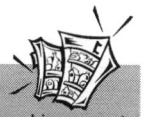

The refrigerator light goes on...
Roasting is an essential technique in cooking great healthy food. The most important thing is that the roasting pan be large enough so that the food doesn't touch. If you use too small a pan, the food will steam and not have that crispy outside the makes roasted food so great.

Nutrition Facts	
Serving size	1 cup
Servings	2
Calories 44	Calories from Fat 10
	% Daily Value
Total Fat 1 g	2 %
Saturated Fat 1 g	3 %
Trans Fat 0 g	
Monounsaturated Fat 0 g	
Cholesterol 2 mg	1 %
Sodium 210 mg	9 %
Total Carbohydrates 8 g	3 %
Dietary Fiber 2 g	9 %
Sugars 6 g	
Protein 1 g	
Vitamin A 2 %	Vitamin C 7 %
Calcium 1 %	Iron 4 %
Vitamin K 0 mcg	
Potassium 269 mg	
Magnesium 19 mg	

Roasted Acorn Squash

Servings = 2
Serving size = 1/2 squash

This recipe can be easily multiplied. The leftovers make a good ingredient in tossed salads.

1	acorn squash (about 1 pound)
1 tsp.	butter
2 tsp.	brown sugar

Preheat oven to 400°F.

Halve the squash lengthwise. Scoop out the seeds and discard them. Make shallow cuts in a grid pattern along the inside of the squash.

Place 1/2 tsp. butter and 1/2 tsp. brown sugar in the cavity of each squash.

Set the squash in the preheated oven and reduce the heat to 350°F. Roast for approximately 30 minutes. Using a spoon occasionally baste the top and inside of the squash with the sugar/butter mixture.

Remove and serve after allowing to cool for about 5 minutes.

"Many so-called aphrodisiac recipes are basically wholesome ingredients prepared in a tasty way. The receptivity to romance probably comes from the general sense of relaxation and well-being good food induces."

Harry E. Wedeck, Author, The Dictionary of Pagan Religions

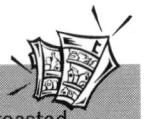

The refrigerator light goes on...
Simple dishes are the best. Pair this roasted acorn squash with a roasted salmon dish and you have the nearly perfect meal.

Nutrition Facts	
Serving size	1/2 squash
Servings	2
Calories 112	Calories from Fat 19
	% Daily Value
Total Fat 2 g	3 %
Saturated Fat 1 g	6 %
Trans Fat 0 g	
Monounsaturated Fat 1 g	
Cholesterol 5 mg	2 %
Sodium 8 mg	0 %
Total Carbohydrates 25 g	8 %
Dietary Fiber 3 g	13 %
Sugars 2 g	
Protein 2 g	
Vitamin A 17 %	Vitamin C 40 %
Calcium 7 %	Iron 9 %
Vitamin K 0 mcg	
Potassium 756 mg	
Magnesium 70 mg	

Brown Rice

Servings = 2
Serving size = 1/2 cup rice

This recipe can easily be multiplied by 2, 3 or 4.
The rice doesn't keep well.

2 1/4 cups	water
1/4 tsp.	salt
1/2 cup	long grain brown rice

In a medium sauce pan, heat the water and salt. When the water boils, stir in the brown rice.

Reduce heat to medium-low and simmer, partially covered, for about 15 minutes.

Do not boil away all of the liquid and do not stir the rice.

When a very small amount of liquid remains, remove the pan from the burner and let it stand, covered, for 5 minutes before serving.

"Rice is the best, the most nutritive and unquestionably the most widespread staple in the world."

Auguste Escoffier, 19th century
French chef

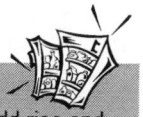

The refrigerator light goes on...
Simple, simple, simple... When you add rice and salt to water and simmer and you don't stir the result is perfect.

Nutrition Facts	
Serving size	about 1/2 cup cooked rice
Servings	2
Calories 171	Calories from Fat 11
	% Daily Value
Total Fat 1 g	2 %
Saturated Fat 0 g	1 %
Trans Fat 0 g	
Monounsaturated Fat 0 g	
Cholesterol 0 mg	0 %
Sodium 294 mg	12 %
Total Carbohydrates 36 g	12 %
Dietary Fiber 2 g	6 %
Sugars 0 g	
Protein 3 g	
Vitamin A 0 %	Vitamin C 0 %
Calcium 1 %	Iron 4 %
Vitamin K 0 mcg	
Potassium 103 mg	
Magnesium 66 mg	

Plain Mashed Potatoes

Servings = 4
Serving size = about one cup

This recipe can easily be multiplied by 2 or 3.
These do not keep very well.

3 quarts	water
1 lb.	yukon gold potatoes
2 tsp.	unsalted butter
1/4 cup	non-fat buttermilk
1/4 cup	2 % milk
1/4 tsp.	salt
to taste	fresh ground black pepper

Place the water in a large stock pot over high heat.

Quarter the potatoes and add to the stock pot. Cover with water by about an inch. Bring to boil and then reduce heat until the water is simmering.

Cook the potatoes about 15 – 20 minutes until slightly soft in the middle. They should give when squeezed.

Remove from heat and drain water. Add butter, buttermilk, milk and salt. Mash potatoes until creamy. I like to leave some chunks. If you like them smooth be careful because over mashing will result in pasty potatoes. Add ground black pepper to taste.

"One potato, two potato, three potato, four."
Child's rhyme

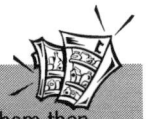

The refrigerator light goes on...
These potatoes have more butter in them than some of the other "flavored" mashed potato recipes in this book. This is to help enhance the creaminess and the mouthfeel that other flavors like roasted garlic or pesto achieve with less fat.

Nutrition Facts	
Serving size	1 cup
Servings	4
Calories 119	Calories from Fat 21
	% Daily Value
Total Fat 2 g	4 %
Saturated Fat 2 g	8 %
Trans Fat 0 g	
Monounsaturated Fat 0 g	
Cholesterol 7 mg	2 %
Sodium 178 mg	7 %
Total Carbohydrates 21 g	7 %
Dietary Fiber 3 g	10 %
Sugars 2 g	
Protein 3 g	
Vitamin A 1 %	Vitamin C 38 %
Calcium 5 %	Iron 5 %
Vitamin K 2 mcg	
Potassium 532 mg	
Magnesium 30 mg	

Roasted Corn on the Cob

Servings = 2
Serving size = 1 ear corn

This recipe is easily multiplied. I love leftover corn. Leave it wrapped in the husks inside the foil.

2 ears	corn
1/8 tsp.	pepper
1/4 tsp.	salt
2 tsp.	unsalted butter

Preheat the oven to 400°F.

Peel the husk back from the corn, being careful not to detach them from the stem. Remove silks and rinse well, wetting down the husks.

Sprinkle the salt and pepper over the corn.

Fold the husks against the corn and wrap in foil.

Roast in the oven for about 30 minutes. Turn them 1/4 turn about every 7 – 8 minutes.

Remove from the oven and unwrap the foil. Cut the bottom of the cob so that the husks fall away easily.

Serve each with a pat of butter.

These can also be roasted on top of the grill. The heat should be medium to medium-high and you must turn them frequently, as noted above.

"The greatest drawback is the way in which it is necessary to eat it. It looks awkward enough: but what is to be done? Surrendering such a vegetable from considerations of grace is not to be thought of."

Harriet Martineau, an Englishwoman writing about corn on the cob in 1835

The refrigerator light goes on...
This recipe includes the pat of butter for your corn on the cob because it just wouldn't be corn without it. Take the pat and enjoy it. This recipe works well both on the grill and in the oven. The grill will give the corn a lovely charcoal flavor.

Nutrition Facts	
Serving size	1 ear
Servings	2
Calories 144	Calories from Fat 44
	% Daily Value
Total Fat 5 g	8 %
Saturated Fat 3 g	13 %
Trans Fat 0 g	
Monounsaturated Fat 1 g	
Cholesterol 10 mg	3 %
Sodium 230 mg	13 %
Total Carbohydrates 26 g	9 %
Dietary Fiber 3 g	11 %
Sugars 4 g	
Protein 3 g	
Vitamin A 2 %	Vitamin C 11 %
Calcium 0 %	Iron 4 %
Vitamin K 1 mcg	
Potassium 258 mg	
Magnesium 33 mg	

Parmesan Squash

Servings = 2
Serving size = 1 large squash

This recipe can easily be multiplied by 2 or 3.
This recipe does not make very good leftovers.

2 large (8 ounces each)	yellow squash
2 cups	water
to taste	fresh ground black pepper
2 Tbsp.	fresh herbs of your choice (minced)
1 oz.	Parmigiano-reggiano (grated)

Place the water in a medium pot fitted with a steamer basket over high heat.

Preheat the oven to 325°F.

Cut about 1/4 inch from the stem end of the squash and then slice lengthwise. Place the four halves in the steamer and steam until slightly tender.

Remove the steamed squash and place in a shallow baking dish. Place the dish in the oven and cook for about 10 minutes. Remove and sprinkle with pepper, fresh herbs and equal amounts of Parmigiano-reggiano.

Return the pan to the oven and cook until the parmesan is melted (about 5 minutes).

"There's no sauce in the world like hunger."
Miguel de Cervantes, Author

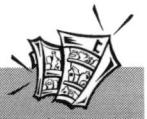

The refrigerator light goes on...
These are two perfect ingredients that make a wonderful dish. The yellow squash tastes like summer and its own buttery flavor is enhanced by the parmesan. I especially like using just a little bit of rosemary for the herb.

Nutrition Facts	
Serving size	1 large squash
Servings	2
Calories 99	Calories from Fat 37
	% Daily Value
Total Fat 4 g	7 %
Saturated Fat 2 g	112 %
Trans Fat 0 g	
Monounsaturated Fat 1 g	
Cholesterol 10 mg	3 %
Sodium 233 mg	10 %
Total Carbohydrates 10 g	3 %
Dietary Fiber 4 g	17 %
Sugars 0 g	
Protein 7 g	
Vitamin A 8 %	Vitamin C 32 %
Calcium 22 %	Iron 7 %
Vitamin K 0 mcg	
Potassium 497 mg	
Magnesium 54 mg	

Melon Salsa

Servings = 8
Serving Size = 1/4 cup
Makes 2 cups

This recipe can be halved or multiplied by 2 or 3.
Keeps in the refrigerator for 24 hours at the most.

6 oz.	cantaloupe (diced)
4 oz.	honeydew melon (diced)
1/4 cup	red onion (diced)
1/4 cup	fresh cilantro (chopped)
1 Tbsp.	fresh lime juice
1/8 tsp.	salt
1/8 tsp.	chili powder

Fold together the cantaloupe, honeydew, red onion, cilantro, lime juice, salt and chili powder.

Chill at least 4 hours.

"If food is poetry, is not poetry also food?"
Joyce Carol Oates, Author

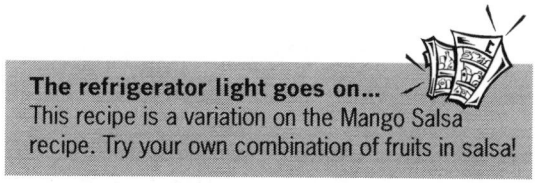

The refrigerator light goes on...
This recipe is a variation on the Mango Salsa recipe. Try your own combination of fruits in salsa!

Nutrition Facts	
Serving size	1/4 cup
Servings	8
Calories 15	Calories from Fat 0
	% Daily Value
Total Fat 0 g	0 %
Saturated Fat 0 g	0 %
Trans Fat 0 g	
Monounsaturated Fat 0 g	
Cholesterol 0 mg	0 %
Sodium 42 mg	2 %
Total Carbohydrates 4 g	1 %
Dietary Fiber 0 g	2 %
Sugars 3 g	
Protein 0 g	
Vitamin A 15 %	Vitamin C 19 %
Calcium 0 %	Iron 1 %
Vitamin K 3 mcg	
Potassium 101 mg	
Magnesium 5 mg	

Couscous

Servings = 4
Serving size = about 1/2 cup

This recipe can easily be multiplied or divided by 2. Keeps well for about 48 hours.

2 cups	water
1/4 tsp.	salt
1 cup	couscous
1 tsp.	olive oil
1/2 cup	dried currants
1	green onion (minced)
1 Tbsp.	flat leaf parsley (chopped fine)
1 Tbsp.	fresh basil (chopped fine)

Place water and salt in a medium sized pan over high heat and bring to a boil. Remove from the heat and add couscous, stirring once. Cover and let stand for five minutes.

As the couscous is cooking, place the oil in a small non-stick sauté pan over medium heat. Add the currants and green onion. Cook, stirring occasionally.

After the couscous has stood for five minutes, remove the top and fluff with a fork. Add the currant and green onion mixture, parsley and basil and toss well.

"Let your food be your medicine, and your medicine be your food."

Hippocrates, Greek physician

The refrigerator light goes on...
Couscous is the perfect pantry item. It keeps almost forever. It is simple to make, taking all of 5 minutes to cook and you can put almost anything in it to make it exotic.

Nutrition Facts	
Serving size	1/2 cup
Servings	4
Calories 225	Calories from Fat 13
	% Daily Value
Total Fat 1 g	2 %
Saturated Fat 0 g	1 %
Trans Fat 0 g	
Monounsaturated Fat 1 g	
Cholesterol 0 mg	0 %
Sodium 152 mg	6 %
Total Carbohydrates 47 g	16 %
Dietary Fiber 4 g	14 %
Sugars 12 g	
Protein 6 g	
Vitamin A 3 %	Vitamin C 5 %
Calcium 3 %	Iron 7 %
Vitamin K 27 mcg	
Potassium 251 mg	
Magnesium 28 mg	

Rice and Lentil Pilaf

Servings = 2
Serving size = about 2 cups.

This recipe can easily be multiplied by 2 or 3.
This recipe keeps well in the refrigerator. Reheat gently.

1 quart	water
1/4 cup	lentils
1 cup	water
1/4 cup	jasmine or basmati rice
1 tsp.	sesame oil
1 small	onion (diced)
1 small (4 ounce)	zucchini (cut into large dice)
1/4 tsp.	salt
to taste	fresh ground black pepper
1/2 tsp.	dried oregano

Place the water in a large stock pot over high heat.

Add the lentils ad cook over a moderate boil for about 25 minutes. Check the degree of doneness about every 3 minutes after 20 minutes and cook until just tender.

While the lentils are cooking place the 1 cup water in a small sauce pan over high heat and bring to a boil. Add the rice and cover. Reduce the heat until the rice is at a simmer. Cook for about 20 - 25 minutes until the water has evaporated and remove from the heat. Keep covered.

While the rice and lentils are cooking place the sesame oil in a medium non-stick skillet over medium heat and add the onions. Cook slowly until they begin to soften. Increase the heat to medium-high and add the zucchini, salt, pepper and oregano. Cook, tossing frequently, until the zucchini begins to brown on all sides.

Drain the cooked lentils well and add to the zucchini. Add the cooked rice to the zucchini and lentils and stir until well blended. Serve.

"If thou tastest a crust of bread, thou tastest all the stars and all the heavens."

Robert Browning, Poet

The refrigerator light goes on...
I know that this recipe uses three pans. There are recipes for pilaf that are one pot and they work OK but I have found that cooking the lentils separate from the rice and veggies keeps the flavors fresher and more distinct. The clean up is not too much problem – all three pans wipe clean with just a bit of soap and water.

Nutrition Facts	
Serving size	about 2 cups
Servings	2
Calories 218	Calories from Fat 25
	% Daily Value
Total Fat 3 g	4 %
Saturated Fat 0 g	2 %
Trans Fat 0 g	
Monounsaturated Fat 1 g	
Cholesterol 0 mg	0 %
Sodium 301 mg	13 %
Total Carbohydrates 40 g	13 %
Dietary Fiber 9 g	37 %
Sugars 4 g	
Protein 9 g	
Vitamin A 3 %	Vitamin C 24 %
Calcium 4 %	Iron 18 %
Vitamin K 6 mcg	
Potassium 478 mg	
Magnesium 50 mg	

Dirty Rice

Servings = 4
Serving size = 1/2 cup rice

This recipe can easily be multiplied by 2, 3 or 4.
The rice doesn't keep well.

1/2 tsp.	chili oil
1/2 tsp.	canola oil
1/4 cup	shallots (minced)
1 1/2 cup	water
1/4 tsp.	salt
1 cup	jasmine rice
1/4 tsp.	ground cumin

Heat the oils over medium heat in a small non-stick skillet. Add the shallots and cook, stirring occasionally. As the shallots cook, increase the heat as needed, so that the shallots brown slightly. When cooked, set aside.

In a medium sauce pan, heat the water and salt. When the liquid boils, stir in the jasmine rice.

Reduce heat to medium-low and simmer, covered, for about 15 minutes.

Do not boil away all of the liquid and do not stir the rice.

When a very small amount of liquid remains, remove the pan from the burner and let it stand, covered, for 3 minutes before serving and then stir in the cooked shallots and the cumin.

"Respect Your Dinner: idolize it, enjoy it properly. You will be many hours in the week, many weeks in the year, and many years in your life happier if you do."

William Makepeace
Thackeray, Author

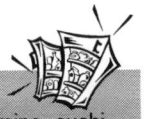

The refrigerator light goes on...
If you haven't noticed, I love rice. Jasmine, sushi, brown, long grained, short grained, risotto – it doesn't matter. You can make rice dirty any way you like. Use whatever leftover veggies that you have. Celery, carrots, peppers, onions, mushrooms will all work well. If you want the rice less spicy, use grapeseed oil instead of the chili oil.

Nutrition Facts	
Serving size about 1/2 cups cooked rice	
Servings	2
Calories 181	Calories from Fat 8
	% Daily Value
Total Fat 1 g	1 %
Saturated Fat 0 g	1 %
Trans Fat 0 g	
Monounsaturated Fat 0 g	
Cholesterol 0 mg	0 %
Sodium 79 mg	3 %
Total Carbohydrates 39 g	13 %
Dietary Fiber 1 g	2 %
Sugars 0 g	
Protein 4 g	
Vitamin A 2 %	Vitamin C 1 %
Calcium 2 %	Iron 12 %
Vitamin K 1 mcg	
Potassium 89 mg	
Magnesium 14 mg	

Mashed Yams

Servings = 4
Serving size = about one cup.

This recipe can easily be multiplied by 2 or 3.
This recipe makes good leftovers and will keep well in the refrigerator for about 48 hours. Reheat gently.

1 quart	water
1 lb.	yams (peeled and cubed)
1 tsp.	extra virgin olive oil
1 large	shallot (minced)
1/4 tsp.	dried rosemary
1/4 tsp.	salt
to taste	fresh ground black pepper
2 Tbsp.	light spread like Take Control or Promise
1/4 cup	non-fat buttermilk
2 Tbsp.	2% milk

Place the water in a large stock pot fitted with a steamer basket over high heat.

Add the cubed yams to the steamer basket and steam until they break slightly with a fork.

While the yams are cooking place the olive oil in a small skillet over medium heat. Add the shallots and rosemary and cook gently until the shallots are softened.

Place the cooked yams together with the shallot and rosemary mixture in a bowl. Add the salt, pepper, spread and buttermilk and mash with a fork until smooth. Add the 2% milk slowly as the yams are mashed smooth.

The mashed yams can be reheated gently in a microwave.

Strange to see how a good dinner and feasting reconciles everybody"

Samuel Pepys, Culinarian

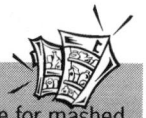

The refrigerator light goes on...
This is the perfect recipe to substitute for mashed potatoes. The same creamy mashed potato dish that's so comforting with the twist of added flavor. And the added benefit of more fiber!

Nutrition Facts	
Serving size	1 cup
Servings	4
Calories 188	Calories from Fat 37
	% Daily Value
Total Fat 4 g	6 %
Saturated Fat 1 g	5 %
Trans Fat 0 g	
Monounsaturated Fat 2 g	
Cholesterol 1mg	0 %
Sodium 215 mg	9 %
Total Carbohydrates 35 g	12 %
Dietary Fiber 5 g	19 %
Sugars 2 g	
Protein 3 g	
Vitamin A 14 %	Vitamin C 35 %
Calcium 6 %	Iron 4 %
Vitamin K 6 mcg	
Potassium 1021 mg	
Magnesium 31 mg	

Zucchini with Sun Dried Tomatoes

Servings = 2
Serving size = about 1 1/2 cups.

This recipe can easily be multiplied by 2, 3, 4, 5, 6, 7, 8. This recipe does not make very good leftovers.

1 tsp.	olive oil
2 medium	sun dried tomato slices
1 Tbsp.	pinenuts
2 medium	zucchini (large dice)
1/4 tsp.	salt
1/4 tsp.	dried thyme leaves
to taste	fresh ground black pepper

Place a large skillet over medium heat. Add the olive oil and after about a minute add the sun dried tomato and pinenuts.

Cook, stirring frequently, for about 5 minutes. Reduce the heat if necessary so that the pinenuts don't brown too much -- they should be a light golden brown.

Add the zucchini, salt, thyme and pepper. Increase the heat to medium high. Cook, tossing frequently, until the zucchini just begins to brown on all sides and is slightly soft.

"Human beings, vegetables, or comic dust, we all dance to a mysterious tune, intoned in the distance by an invisible player,"

Albert Einstein, Physicist

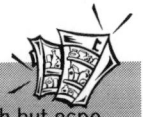

The refrigerator light goes on...
This goes so well with almost any dish but especially a steak or roasted pork main course. The zucchini is simple to prep. Cut the stem end off and make three slices lengthways so you have 4 slices. Stack two slices and cut lengthways three times again. Do this with all four slices and then cut crossways for a large dice.

Nutrition Facts	
Serving size	1 1/2 cups
Servings	4
Calories 84	Calories from Fat 47
	% Daily Value
Total Fat 5 g	8 %
Saturated Fat 1 g	3 %
Trans Fat 0 g	
Monounsaturated Fat 2 g	
Cholesterol 0 mg	0 %
Sodium 352 mg	15 %
Total Carbohydrates 8 g	3 %
Dietary Fiber 3 g	10 %
Sugars 4 g	
Protein 3 g	
Vitamin A 8 %	Vitamin C 57 %
Calcium 3 %	Iron 7 %
Vitamin K 15 mcg	
Potassium 607 mg	
Magnesium 47 mg	

Thick Cut Yam Fries

Servings = 2
Serving size = about 1 1/2 cups fries

This recipe can easily be multiplied by 2, 3, 4, 5, 6, 7, 8. This recipe does not make very good leftovers.

2 small	yams (about 5 ounces each)
1/4 tsp.	salt
to taste	fresh ground black pepper
1/8 tsp.	dried thyme leaves
	spray olive oil

Place a large skillet in the oven and set the preheat to 325°F.

Scrub the yams well and then cut into wedges. It's easiest to cut them in half lengthwise and then quarters and then eighths.

When the oven is hot spray the pan lightly with oil. Add the yam wedges and sprinkle the salt, pepper and thyme over the top. Spray lightly with olive oil.

Return the pan to the oven and cook for about 25 minutes tossing frequently.

Serve hot.

"If life were fair, Dan Quayle would be making a living asking 'Do you want fries with that?"
John Cleese, Genius

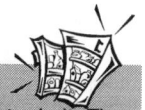

The refrigerator light goes on...
This recipe is so simple you just have to do it. The prep takes all of two minutes. Tossing them into a pan and watching them another 20 minutes. Great fries to go with that Turkey Burger in 25-30 minutes total. Easy!

Nutrition Facts	
Serving size	about 1/2 cups fries
Servings	2
Calories 185	Calories from Fat 22
	% Daily Value
Total Fat 2 g	4 %
Saturated Fat 0 g	2 %
Trans Fat 0 g	
Monounsaturated Fat 0 g	
Cholesterol 0 mg	0 %
Sodium 303 mg	13 %
Total Carbohydrates 39 g	13 %
Dietary Fiber 6 g	23 %
Sugars 1 g	
Protein 2 g	
Vitamin A 4 %	Vitamin C 40 %
Calcium 3 %	Iron 5 %
Vitamin K 6 mcg	
Potassium 1143 mg	
Magnesium 30 mg	

Beef Stew

Servings = 6
Serving size = 2 1/2 cups

I would not multiply this recipe but it can be halved. Leftovers are better than fresh.

4 cups	water
25	pearl onions (peeled)
1/3 cup	all purpose flour
1 tsp.	salt
1/4 tsp.	fresh ground black pepper
1 1/2 Lbs.	flank steak (3/4 inch cubes)
	cooking spray
1/2 lb.	button mushrooms (quartered)
1 cup	white onion (sliced)
1 Tbsp.	lemon juice
1 Tbsp.	Worcestershire sauce
1 lb.	carrots (peeled & sliced 1/4 inch thick)
2	bay leaves
1 1/2 Lbs.	red potatoes (cut into 3/4 inch cubes)
1/8 tsp.	ground allspice
4 cups	water

Heat water in a medium stockpot over high heat until it is at a shiver. Add pearl onions and cook for about ten minutes. Drain and place the onions in a large stock pot.

Preheat oven to 400°F.

Mix flour, salt and pepper in a paper bag. Toss the cubes of flank steak in the flour, coating well.

Coat a large skillet with cooking spray and heat over medium-high heat. Add cubes of flank steak and cook, turning until all sides are brown. Do not over-crowd the beef or the meat will steam and not brown. Remove the meat to the stock pot as it browns.

Add the onions to the skillet and cook until they are soft and brown. Add them to the stock pot.
Add the lemon juice and Worcestershire sauce to the skillet and deglaze the pan, scraping up anything stuck to the bottom of the pan. Add the deglazing liquid to the stock pot.

Add carrots, bay leaves, potatoes, allspice and water to the stock-pot.

Place covered pot in the oven and reduce heat to 400°F. Cook for one hour stirring gently every fifteen minutes.

"The most remarkable thing about my mother is that for thirty years she served the family nothing but leftovers. The original meal has never been found."

Calvin Trillin, Epicurean author

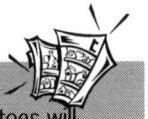

The refrigerator light goes on...
Don't stir stews too often or the potatoes will break down. Gently stir the stew, at most, about every 15 minutes.

Nutrition Facts	
Serving size	about 2 1/2 cups
Servings	8
Calories 356	Calories from Fat 69
	% Daily Value
Total Fat 8 g	12 %
Saturated Fat 3 g	15 %
Trans Fat 0 g	
Monounsaturated Fat 3 g	
Cholesterol 47 mg	16 %
Sodium 544 mg	23 %
Total Carbohydrates 43 g	14 %
Dietary Fiber 6 g	26 %
Sugars 10 g	
Protein 30 g	
Vitamin A 251 %	Vitamin C 41 %
Calcium 10 %	Iron 21 %
Vitamin K 15 mcg	
Potassium 1445 mg	
Magnesium 76 mg	

Minestrone

8 60 min.

(requires overnight soaking of beans)
Serving size = about 2 cups

This keeps well for about 4 days in the fridge. Reheat gently. Serve with a side salad of your choice.

1 lb.	great northern beans
2 quarts	water
2 tsp.	olive oil
3 cloves	garlic (minced)
2 cups	onion (diced)
1/2 lb.	parsnips (peeled and sliced)
1/2 lb.	carrots (peeled and sliced)
3 ribs	celery (sliced)
4 cups	water
Rind (about 3" x 3")	Parmigiano-Reggiano
3	bay leaves
4 cups	non fat chicken stock
1 1/2 lbs.	red potatoes (peeled and cubed)
2 - 28 oz. cans	peeled whole tomatoes (drain & seed tomatoes)
1/2 tsp.	salt
1 Tbsp. (per serving)	flat leaf parsley (minced)
1 Tbsp. (per serving)	Parmigiano-Reggiano (grated)

Rinse beans thoroughly.

Cover beans with water and allow to soak overnight. Drain and rinse. Place in a stock pot and add two quarts water to cover.

Simmer over medium heat for 30 - 45 minutes until the beans just begin to turn soft. Drain.

While the beans are cooking heat oil in a large stock pot over medium. Add the minced garlic. Cook garlic in oil slowly. Do not allow this to brown or the garlic will become bitter. Add onion and cook slowly until it just begins to turn soft.

Add the parsnips, carrots and celery and cook over medium-low heat until the vegetables begin to soften. Cover with the water and chicken stock and add the potatoes and the rind of parmesan. Cook over medium-low heat for about 20 minutes until the potatoes begin to soften. Add the tomatoes, beans and salt. Cook for about 20 minutes and remove the rind of parmesan.

Serve each 2 cup serving with 1 tablespoon minced parsley and grated parmesan. As with most soups this one is best made the day in advance.

"To feel safe and warm on a cold wet night, all you really need is soup."

Laurie Colwin, Author

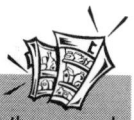

The refrigerator light goes on...
This soup, as with most soups, is best the second or third day. It is so good and so good for you making a batch in the dead of winter to have for dinner and then a few lunches will make you feel so warm. If you are out of an ingredient, that's OK. There are plenty of substitutions. Almost any root vegetable will do.

Nutrition Facts	
Serving size	2 cups
Servings	4
Calories 405	Calories from Fat 51
	% Daily Value
Total Fat 6 g	9 %
Saturated Fat 2 g	12 %
Trans Fat 0 g	
Monounsaturated Fat 2 g	
Cholesterol 7 mg	2 %
Sodium 569 mg	24 %
Total Carbohydrates 70 g	23 %
Dietary Fiber 18 g	71 %
Sugars 12 g	
Protein 23 g	
Vitamin A 107 %	Vitamin C 71 %
Calcium 33 %	Iron 36 %
Vitamin K 88 mcg	
Potassium 1935 mg	
Magnesium 170 mg	

Split Pea Soup

4 60 min.

Serving size = about two cups.

This recipe can easily be multiplied by 2. This recipe is better the next day. Store tightly covered in the refrigerator.

Serve with a 2 ounce whole grain roll and a side salad of your choice.

2 quarts	water
1 cup	split peas
1 tsp.	grapeseed oil
2 oz.	prosciutto ham (diced)
1 medium	onion (diced)
6 cups	water
1/2 tsp.	salt
to taste	fresh ground black pepper
1/4 tsp	ground nutmeg
2 Tbsp.	dry sherry

Place the split peas in the boiling water and cook at a rolling boil for 2 minutes and remove from heat. Let stand for an hour and drain.

Place the grapeseed oil in a 4 quart sauce pan over medium heat. Add the diced ham and cook slowly until the ham is not quite crispy. This will take about 5 minutes.

Add the onion and increase the heat slightly. Cook, stirring frequently, until the onions begin to be soft. Add the split peas and stir well.

Add the water and salt and cook for about an hour over low-medium heat. Stir occasionally.

When the split peas are slightly soft to your taste remove the pan from the heat. Remove about 1 1/2 cups of the soup and puree the remaining using a stick blender or blender. Add the 1 1/2 cups of split peas back to the soup and stir.

Add the nutmeg and sherry and cook for another 5 minutes.

"I live on good soup, not on fine words."
Moliere, Author

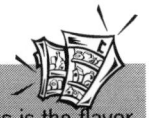

The refrigerator light goes on...
I loved split pea soup as a kid and this is the flavor that I have been craving for some time. I don't really know why I didn't work on this recipe years ago. It is easier to soak the beans overnight and then you don't have to boil them and let them stand for an hour. Simply soak overnight, drain, use.

Nutrition Facts	
Serving size	2 cups
Servings	4
Calories 226	Calories from Fat 26
	% Daily Value
Total Fat 3 g	5 %
Saturated Fat 1 g	3 %
Trans Fat 0 g	
Monounsaturated Fat 1 g	
Cholesterol 8 mg	3 %
Sodium 483 mg	20 %
Total Carbohydrates 34 g	11 %
Dietary Fiber 13 g	53 %
Sugars 6 g	
Protein 15 g	
Vitamin A 1 %	Vitamin C 6 %
Calcium 4 %	Iron 13 %
Vitamin K 7 mcg	
Potassium 577 mg	
Magnesium 64 mg	

Creamy Chicken and Potato Soup

4 60 min.

Serving size = about 2 cups

This recipe can easily be multiplied by 2. As with almost all soups this recipe is better the next day.

2 tsp.	grapeseed or olive oil
1 large	red onion (diced)
2 large	carrots (peeled and diced)
1 clove	garlic (minced)
2 cups	low-sodium chicken stock
1/2 cup	water
1/4 tsp.	salt
1 lb.	Yukon gold potatoes (cut into 1 inch cubes)
to taste	fresh ground black pepper
1 lb.	boneless chicken breast (cut into 1/2 inch cubes)
1 cup	2% milk
3 Tbsp.	fresh dill

Place the grapeseed oil in a large stock pot over medium heat. Add the red onion and cook for about 3 minutes.

Add the carrots and garlic and cook for another 5 minutes until the onions begin to turn translucent.

Add the chicken stock, water, salt and potatoes. Season with pepper and reduce the heat to low.

Simmer for about 50 minutes. Stir occasionally. Cook until the potatoes are soft and beginning to fall apart.

Add the chicken breast and fresh dill. Stir and then slowly add the milk. Cook for another ten minutes.

Serve.

"It was a big story and yesterday's soup. Who cares?"

Willard Scott, Weatherman

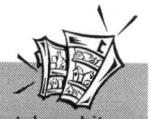

The refrigerator light goes on...
This is a quick and easy soup. It does take a bit of time to simmer – just long enough to watch Jeopardy – but it's perfect on a cold night – warm, creamy and really filling. All of that with 5 grams of fiber and tons of vitamins.

Nutrition Facts	
Serving size	2 cups
Servings	4
Calories 327	Calories from Fat 52
	% Daily Value
Total Fat 6 g	9 %
Saturated Fat 2 g	8 %
Trans Fat 0 g	
Monounsaturated Fat 1 g	
Cholesterol 70 mg	23 %
Sodium 338 mg	14 %
Total Carbohydrates 35 g	12 %
Dietary Fiber 5 g	20 %
Sugars 9 g	
Protein 34 g	
Vitamin A 189 %	Vitamin C 52 %
Calcium 15 %	Iron 13 %
Vitamin K 10 mcg	
Potassium 1228 mg	
Magnesium 80 mg	

Lentil Soup

Servings = 4
Serving size = about 2 cups.

This recipe can easily be multiplied by 2, 3, 4. This recipe is better the second day.

1 Tbsp.	olive oil
1 large	white onion (diced)
2 ribs	celery (diced)
2 large	carrots (peeled and diced)
4 ounces	sliced ham (cut into small dice)
1/2 tsp.	salt
to taste	fresh ground black pepper
1 cup	lentils
1 Tbsp.	dried sage (crumbled)
2	bay leaves
1/2 tsp.	dried thyme leaves
2 cups	low-sodium chicken stock
8 cups	water

Place the olive oil in a large sauce pan over medium heat. Add the onion and cook for about 5 minutes and add the celery and carrots.

Cook, stirring frequently, for about 5 minutes and add the ham.

Cook, stirring frequently, for about 5 minutes and add the salt, pepper, lentils, sage, bay leaves, thyme chicken stock and water.

Stir well and reduce the heat to medium-low Cook for about 45 minutes until the lentils are soft.

"Every leaf speaks bliss to me, fluttering from the autumn tree"

Emily Bronte, Author

The refrigerator light goes on...
This is the perfect soup for autumn. Pair this with a simple side salad and you have the best fall meal going. I look for ham that's as low in sodium as I can find. The Healthy Choice is a pretty good pick but there are a lot of sliced hams on the market that are minimally processed with no nitrates and are much lower in sodium.

Nutrition Facts	
Serving size	2 cups
Servings	4
Calories 296	Calories from Fat 53
	% Daily Value
Total Fat 6 g	9 %
Saturated Fat 1 g	6 %
Trans Fat 0 g	
Monounsaturated Fat 3 g	
Cholesterol 41 mg	14 %
Sodium 699 mg	29 %
Total Carbohydrates 41 g	14 %
Dietary Fiber 17 g	70 %
Sugars 6 g	
Protein 21 g	
Vitamin A 189 %	Vitamin C 16 %
Calcium 7 %	Iron 26 %
Vitamin K 21 mcg	
Potassium 938 mg	
Magnesium 80 mg	

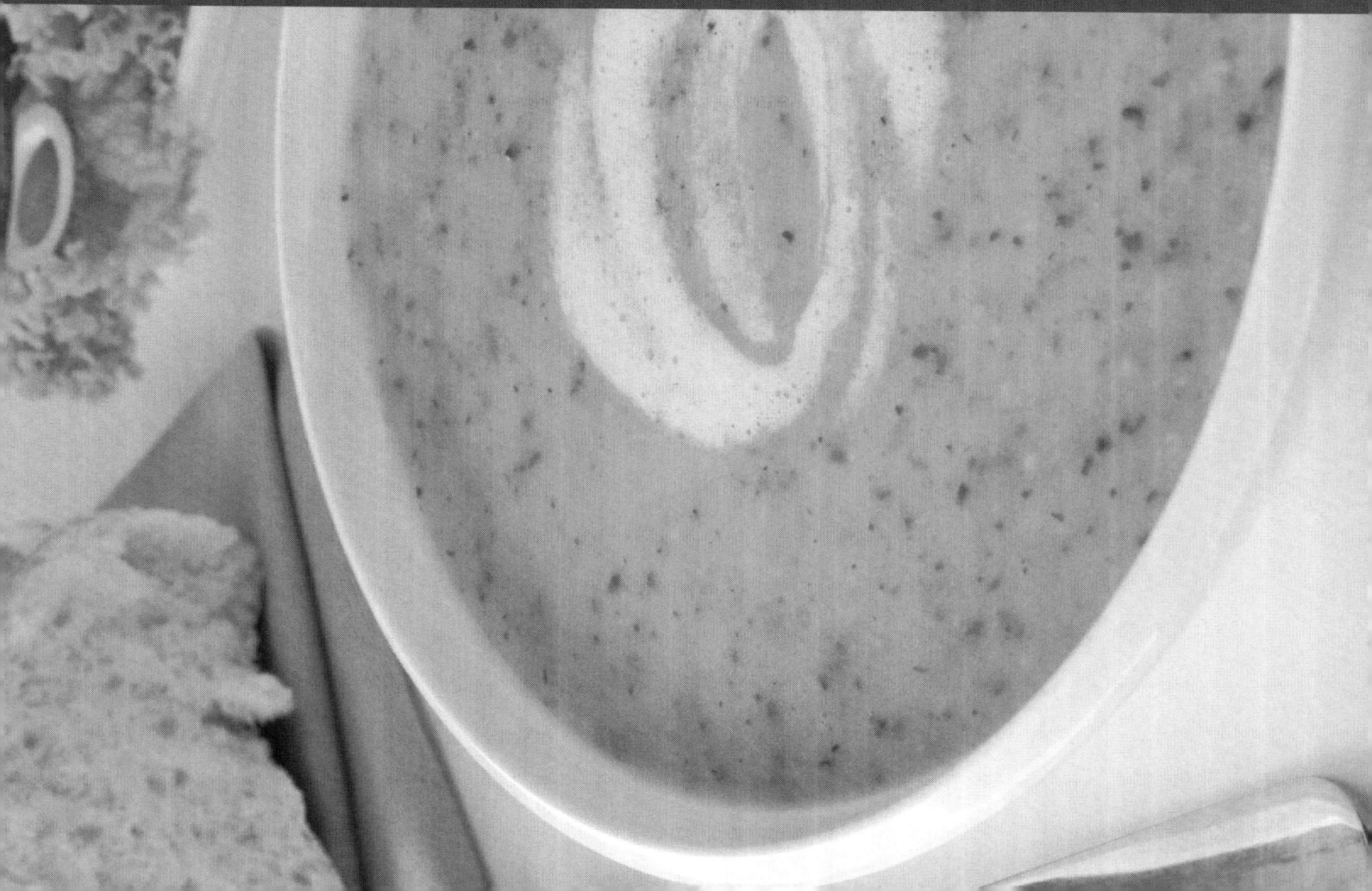

I get lots of questions about Coumadin® (warfarin). Here are some common questions.

Does salt increase INR levels?

My girlfriend (age 46) just had a heart valve replacement and was placed on Coumadin. She was told to avoid food with a high sodium content. We have some questions about this and what actually affect her INR levels.

Does salt actually increase the INR level? They also told her she could use "sea salt" in moderation, but from what I have read it's still salt, is this true? Is sea salt really better for you?

What about the lack of iodine in sea salt, I have not found any iodized sea salt yet. Does she need to worry about iodine supplements if using non-iodized sea salt or salt substitutes?

Dr. Gourmet Says...

The sodium content of table salt (sodium chloride) should not have an effect on your girlfriend's INR or her Coumadin® (warfarin). It may be that her doctor wanted to make sure that there are no problems with salt worsening her high blood pressure or issues of fluid overload in the body that could lead to Congestive Heart Failure (CHF).

Sea salt is salt. A teaspoon might have a little less sodium in it because of the fact that sea salt crystals are larger and therefore don't stack together in a spoon like Morton's salt. That said, salt is salt. There are impurities in sea salt that can contribute to flavors in the salt, but otherwise the sodium and chloride are the same. Sea salt is salt and all salt in excess is something that pretty much everyone should avoid. I don't see that sea salt is worth the extra money.

Most folks get enough iodine in a healthy diet. Using a mixture of salt and sea salt should be fine but check with her doctor about the amount of sodium he wants her to have each day. She really shouldn't need to worry about iodine supplements this way.

Can I cook with parsley while on Coumadin?

I am trying to work out my new diet. The list says 1 cup of raw parsley is very high. Can I use a small amount to cook with?

Dr. Gourmet Says...

I suspect that parsley accounts for more of the variation that physicians and patients find with INR levels in those taking Coumadin® (warfarin).

This is because parsley contains a lot of Vitamin K. The USDA Ingredient Database reports that a tablespoon has 62 micrograms (mcg). This can add up quite fast in a meal that has a couple of tablespoons of parsley as a garnish or in a dressing.

Should I avoid lettuce while on Coumadin?

I was told that if you are on Coumadin you should not eat lettuce. Is this true?

Dr. Gourmet Says...

Because Vitamin K can have an effect on how Coumadin® (warfarin) is processed in your body it is important to have about the same amounts of Vitamin K each day.

Lettuces are members of the cabbage family. As a rule cabbages contain higher amounts of Vitamin K. Part of eating healthy is to eat a lot of green leafy vegetables but this can be a problem for those people who use Coumadin as a result. If you are going to begin eating lettuce and other members of the cabbage family, it is important to be consistent. By that I mean you should eat about the same amount of such green leafy vegetables each day so that your INR doesn't fluctuate.

Take a look at the Vitamin K Levels in Foods list later in this book. Take this to your doctor and discuss eating a consistent serving of such foods. That way the two of you can more closely monitor your INR while you are adapting your diet.

Can you wean down your dose of Coumadin?

Is it possible to increase certain things like Vitamin E, A and C so that you can lower the dose of Coumadin needed? Of course you would have to be monitored by your doctor, but is it possible to use Garlic or some natural ways to thin your blood so you would not have to take so much Coumadin?

I'm a registered nurse and my cousin has to take 30 pills every day, including 10mg of Coumadin. She is asking me if there is any way she could be weaned off of some of the medicine.

Thank you so much for your information. I have printed her your list of foods and their Vitamin K content. Besides lowering her intake of Vitamin K what else can she do to thin her blood?

Dr. Gourmet Says...

I don't know of any research that supports using vitamins or other supplements to reduce the dose of Coumadin® (warfarin). I am not sure how to have your cousin weaned off of any of her medications but often a visit with her doctor to discuss this subject and / or consolidation of some pills is helpful.

There are no clinically proven methods to help "thin" her blood other than the medications recommended by her physician.

Does Coumadin cause fatigue?

My mother is on Coumadin. She is also on Vicodin for pain. She is chronically tired all the time! Is Coumadin a contributing factor for this tiredness? I know that the Vicodin is. Can you help me know what foods she could eat to boost her energy?

Dr. Gourmet Says...

Your question is a common one that I often encounter. Certainly the Vicodin can be a major contributing factor to your mother's fatigue. Using narcotics in the elderly for pain control can be a challenge.

Fatigue is not a common complaint of those using Coumadin® (warfarin), but I have learned in my practice that patients will react to medications in different ways - so it is possible that your mother's tiredness is related. As a physician I always have to ask if there is some medication that I might be prescribing that could cause issues. There are common medications that some take while taking Coumadin that might be involved. These include beta blockers (atenolol, metoprolol, propranolol, etc.), calcium channel blockers (amlodipine, diltiazem) as well as many anti-depressants.

Oftentimes depression can be the culprit and fatigue in the elderly always makes me question if this is an issue. Part of the work up for fatigue and depression include evaluating thyroid function and Vitamin B12 levels. Hemoglobin is key in the work up for fatigue as well. Chat with her about going with her to the next doctor's appointment. Many times our elderly patients will tell their physicians "everything's just fine" when it isn't. I have been told many times by patients, "I just didn't want to bother you with my problems -- you need to take your time with someone who is really sick." (Except, of course, it's your mother who we want to take care of.)

There is a great deal of controversy about whether foods can boost energy or not. Certainly there are thousands of websites purporting that particular foods and diets can provide everything from energy to longevity to boosting the immune system. While much of the research that has been done is encouraging regarding the effect of diet on long term health, most are smaller studies and require more research. Likewise, few have shown specific short term benefits for malaise and fatigue.

That said, I do find diet to often be a concern. A major issue in the elderly can be that they will often not cook fresh foods for themselves and sometimes eat less healthy. Skipping meals can be a major problem, as well as relying on more processed foods and not getting fresh, whole foods. The consequence can be fewer calories than they actually need and the quality of those calories can be lacking.

One strategy is to ask her if you can take a look in her cabinets and fridge. Sometimes the food is there but she might not be eating it. Having your mom keep a food diary can be one path to seeing what she is eating and how often.

Lastly, there are many services that will help provide her with ready made meals. Check with your local grocery about whether they are able to help.

Does Coumadin® (warfarin) affect your metabolism and cause weight gain?

My wife has been taking warfarin for over two months. When she started exercising for three days a week, in a month's time she has gained 12 pounds, and her diet did not change. Before she started exercising she was losing some amount of weight. She will be using warfarin for the next four months. Do you think warfarin has affected her metabolism? If yes how could she lose weight then?

Dr. Gourmet Says...

This is a very interesting question. There is no evidence that Coumadin® (warfarin) leads to weight gain. As a physician my first question would be whether there is a medical issue that is leading to your wife's weight gain. It is important that she discuss this with her doctor. Perhaps there is another medication that she is taking that could lead to weight gain. Some people who take Coumadin for certain heart problems are more susceptible to congestive heart failure and that is the sort of issue her physician would want to know about.

Weight loss is accomplished by eating fewer calories and exercising more. Often people will use supplements like sports drinks and the like while exercising that they feel are healthy but are actually just added calories. Keeping a food diary is a good first step for your wife. This can help her to get an idea of what she is eating. Many times asking one's doctor for a referral to the dietician can help and having the food diary can be an aid to helping create a diet that works for your wife.

Should you avoid cranberry juice on Coumadin® (warfarin)?

My husband may have a kidney infection and I wanted to give him cranberry juice, but he is on Coumadin. Would this affect his medicine?

Dr. Gourmet Says...

Up until recently I would have said that it would be wise to avoid it. A report in the *British Medical Journal* in 2003 was concerning. The patient in question was drinking a great deal of cranberry juice and on an essentially liquid diet. There were other case reports, but no well-designed study that investigated the issue until more recently. The good news is that we now have pretty good evidence that it's OK to drink cranberry juice.

The feeling had been that somehow cranberry juice interacted with the cytochrome P450 system of enzymes, which are critical to helping the body clear itself of chemicals such as medications we take.

A group of researchers in Boston looked at whether cranberry juice, brewed tea, grape juice or placebo would have an effect on the specific P450 enzyme responsible for clearing warfarin from the body. They used another drug, fluconazole, as a control medication. (*Clin Pharmacol Ther* 2006;79:125–33.) No effect was seen on the clearance of medications in the body by any of the test substances.

In another study, a group had ten healthy volunteers drink cranberry juice or water each day for ten days. They tested three different drugs, including warfarin, to see if there was any difference in the drug concentrations or the INR. Again, no difference. (*Clin Pharmacol Ther* 2007;81:833–39.) We were right to be cautious because of the case reports, but now we have evidence that it's OK for you to drink cranberry juice while taking Coumadin (warfarin).

Does alcohol interact with Coumadin?

My mother is taking Coumadin. For years when my brother comes over for Monday night dinner my mom and brother have one shot of Crown Royal. Could my mom have a tiny bite of alchol? If she does, what will happen? She is 91 years old.

Dr. Gourmet Says...

Most physicians deal with alcohol use in their patients on a case by case basis.

The amount of Crown Royal is small enough that it would likely not be a problem for your mom's warfarin use. However, patients who take Coumadin are often on a number of other medications that alcohol can interact with.

Check with her doctor to make sure that he or she feels a drink with your Monday night dinners is OK.

Should I avoid caffeinated coffee on Coumadin® (warfarin)?

I am on Coumadin, do I have to drink Decaf coffee only. If I drink regular coffee, would it give me a headache?

Dr. Gourmet Says...

Many physicians wish for their patients to not consume caffeine. There is scant evidence to support this posture, but many people do feel better drinking coffee or tea with no caffeine. You would need to ask your doctor how he or she feels about this for your case.

Many people who drink a lot of beverages that contain caffeine develop a dependency. When they stop consuming caffeine abruptly they can often have symptoms of fatigue and headache. If you are used to drinking a lot of regular coffee, it might be a good idea for you to taper off slowly, drinking a little less each day for about a week.

One way to do this is to mix regular coffee with decaf before you brew the coffee. Each day use less regular and more decaf in brewing. After a week or so you will be using only decaffeinated.

How much Vitamin K is in Fresca®, Sprite®, or other sodas?

Hello-my father is on Coumadin (almost died of a AAA). We were discussing that his levels fluctuate because of Fresca soda or maybe some Sprite/7Up he drinks. Would this have a major factor on his med. Also when you discuss Cola-does root beer fall in this category.

Dr. Gourmet Says...

The USDA reports that Sprite® contains no Vitamin K at all. Their database doesn't contain information on Fresca® but there is information on many other types of soda. Cola, with or without caffeine as well as with or without sugar, does not have any Vitamin K.

The same is true for cream soda, club soda, ginger ale, grape soda, Dr. Pepper®, orange soda, root beer and tonic water.

It appears that users of Coumadin® (warfarin) would be safe drinking soda. That said, soda is not a good choice for a healthy diet. Drinking a cola or root beer occasionally is fine and one should choose sugar free products. There is plenty of research now that shows how much better other beverages can be for your health. Choose water, juice, tea, coffee or green tea instead.

If I'm on Coumadin, can I use Green Tea for weight loss?

I take 2.5 mg Coumadin 5 days each week for Fibrillation. Is it OK to use Green Tea Supplement drinks to try for some weight control?

Dr. Gourmet Says...

Green tea and green tea supplements have become very popular in the last few years and have been touted as a panacea for many illnesses. While drinking green tea may be beneficial, there is less evidence to support the use of green tea extract, which is often marketed and used for weight loss. While there is some evidence to support this, there may be some risk. In a Clinical Observation published in *The Annals of Internal Medicine* (2006; 144: 68-69), Dr. Herbert Bonkovsky reports on a case of liver toxicity related to green tea extract.

The patient, a 37 year old woman, had arrived at the hospital complaining of abdominal pain, nausea and jaundice. Testing for infection was negative, but a liver biopsy showed liver damage. She had been taking "The Right Approach Complex", a weight loss supplement containing green tea extract. When she stopped taking the supplement, her liver tests returned to normal.

One year later the same patient was admitted to the hospital again with the same symptoms. A month earlier she had started taking the same supplement. Testing of her liver showed similar results to the previous year and again returned to normal after stopping the supplement for the second time. This is what doctors call a "positive rechallenge," meaning that the supplement caused problems with a second use or "challenge." This is generally taken as evidence of a medication or supplement as the cause of a side effect.

While one popular website still reports "To date, the only negative side effect reported from drinking green tea is insomnia due to the fact that it contains caffeine," this is clearly not the case with supplements. Dr. Bonkovsky reports eight other cases where use of green tea extract caused liver problems.

As with all supplements, it is wise to be extremely careful and research them thoroughly before use - or avoid them altogether. Talk with your doctor and let them know if you are using supplements especially if you are using Coumadin® (warfarin) or any other prescription medication as many can not only cause health problems but can also interact with other medications.

Are there any documented problems with people drinking the supplement "Mona Vie" while on Coumadin?

Dr. Gourmet Says...

There are not any significant studies that would lead one to believe that this is anything more than expensive juice. There is no information on interaction with Coumadin® (warfarin) that I am aware of.

Stick to healthy, fresh fruit. Cheaper, more satisfying and proven to be good for you.

Vitamin K Content of Foods

Short list

This is the down and dirty list–one that you can keep on hand so that you know what foods to avoid.

High (over 40 mcg Vitamin K per serving)

Vegetables	Serving Size	mcg per serving
Spinach, frozen	10 oz.	1189.5
Parsley, raw	1 cup	984.0
Spinach, cooked	1 cup	888.5
Collard Greens, cooked	1 cup	836.0
Kale, raw, chopped	1 cup	547.4
Swiss Chard, raw	1 cup	298.8
Mustard greens, raw, chopped	1 cup	278.5
Broccoli, cooked, chopped	1 cup	220.2
Brussels sprouts, cooked	1 cup	218.8
Onions, green/scallions, raw	1 cup	207.0
Brussels sprouts, raw	1 cup	155.8
Spinach, raw	1 cup	144.9
Turnip greens, raw	1 cup	138.1
Endive, raw, chopped	1 cup	115.6
Broccoli, raw, chopped	1 cup	92.5
Watercress, raw	1 cup	85.0
Okra, cooked	1 cup	64.0
Lettuce, green leaf, raw	1 cup	62.5
Peas, green, frozen, cooked	10 oz	60.7
Lettuce, Boston/Bibb, raw	1 cup	56.3
Leek, raw	1 medium	41 8
Lettuce, Romaine, raw	1 cup	48.2
Cabbage, napa, raw, shredded	1 cup	42.0
Peas, green, cooked	1 cup	41.4
Peas, sugar snap, cooked	1 cup	40.0

Legumes and Beans		mcg per serving
Soybeans (edamame)	1 cup	87.4

Misc.		mcg per serving
Cilantro, fresh	9 sprigs	62.0

Medium (between 20 and 40 mcg Vitamin K per serving)

Vegetables	Serving Size	mcg per serving
Lettuce, red leaf, raw	1 cup	39.3
Asparagus, cooked	5 spears	38.0
Spaghetti/Marinara sauce	1 cup	34.8
Asparagus, raw	5 spears	33.5
Cabbage, red, raw, shredded	1 cup	26.7
Lettuce, Iceberg, raw	2 cups	26.6
Cabbage, Chinese, raw, shredded	1 cup	25.1
Tomatoes, sun-dried	1 Cup	23.2
Peas & onions, frozen, cooked	1 cup	21.8
Carrots, cooked, slices	1 cup	21.4
Cauliflower, cooked	1 cup	21.4

Fruits	Serving Size	mcg per serving
Pumpkin, canned	1 cup	39.2
Kiwi fruit	1 medium	30.6
Blackberries	1 cup	28.5
Blueberries	1 cup	28.0
Grapes, red/green, seedless	1 cup	23.4

Legumes and Beans	Serving Size	mcg per serving
Bean sprouts, mung, fresh	1 cup	34.3
Cashews	½ cup	23.8

Misc.	Serving Size	mcg per serving
Thyme, dried	1 tsp	24.0

Comprehensive list

This is nearly a complete list of the foods used in this book and on DrGourmet.com that you can use for reference if you have a question about a particular ingredient.

Vegetables	Serving Size	mcg per serving
Anchovies, fillets	1 each	0.5
Asparagus, raw	5 spears	33.5
Asparagus, cooked	5 spears	38.0
Beans, green, cooked	1 cup	20.0
Beans, yellow (wax beans), raw	1 cup	0.0
Beets, cooked, sliced	1 cup	0.40
Broccoli, raw, chopped	1 cup	92.5
Broccoli, cooked, chopped	1 cup	220.2
Brussels sprouts, cooked	1 cup	218.8
Brussels sprouts, raw	1 cup	155.8
Cabbage, Chinese, raw, shredded	1 cup	25.1
Cabbage, napa, raw, shredded	1 cup	42.0
Cabbage, red, raw, shredded	1 cup	26.7
Carrots, raw, strips or slices	1 cup	16.1
Carrots, cooked, slices	1 cup	21.4
Cauliflower, raw	1 cup	16.0
Cauliflower, cooked	1 cup	21.4
Celery	1 stalk	11.7
Collard Greens, cooked	1 cup	836.0
Corn, yellow, cooked	1 cup	0.7
Corn, yellow, raw	1 cup	0.5
Cucumber	1 medium	14.5
Eggplant, raw, cubed	1 cup	2.9
Eggplant, cooked, cubed	1 cup	2.9
Endive, raw, chopped	1 cup	115.6
Fennel	1 bulb	0
Garlic	3 cloves	0.1
Kale, raw, chopped	1 cup	547.4
Leek, raw	1 medium	41
8Lettuce, arugula	1/2 cup	10.9
Lettuce, Boston/Bibb, raw	1 cup	56.3
Lettuce, green leaf, raw	1 cup	62.5
Lettuce, red leaf, raw	1 cup	39.3
Lettuce, Romaine, raw	1 cup	48.2
Lettuce, Iceberg, raw	1 cup	13.3
Mushrooms, raw	1 cup	0
Mustard greens, raw, chopped	1 cup	278.5
Okra, cooked	1 cup	64.0
Onions, green/scallions, raw	1 cup	207.0

Onions, white/red/yellow, raw	1 cup	0.6
Parsley, raw	1 cup	984.0
Parsnips, cooked	1 cup	1.6
Peas, green, frozen, cooked	10 oz	60.7
Peas, green, cooked	1 cup	41.4
Peas & onions, frozen, cooked	1 cup	21.8
Peas, sugar snap, cooked	1 cup	40.0
Pepper, green bell	1 medium	8.8
Pepper, jalapeno	1 medium	1.4
Pepper, red bell	1 medium	5.8
Pepper, red chili, hot	1 each	6.3
Pepper, yellow sweet	1medium	0
Potato, red, cooked	1 medium	4.8
Potato, white, baked	1 medium	4.7
Potato, sweet, cooked	1 medium	2.6
Shallots, chopped	1 Tbsp	0
Snow peas, raw	1 cup	15.8
Spaghetti/Marinara sauce	1 cup	34.8
Spinach, raw	1 cup	144.9
Spinach, cooked	1 cup	888.5
Spinach, frozen	10 oz.	1189.5
Squash, acorn	1 cup	0
Squash, butternut, cooked, cubed	1 cup	2.0
Squash, summer, cooked	1 cup	6.3
Swiss Chard, raw	1 cup	298.8
Tomato paste	1 Tbsp	1.8
Tomato, plum	1	4.9
Tomato, raw	1 medium	9.7
Tomato sauce, canned, no salt	1 cup	6.8
Tomatoes, canned, whole	1 cup	7.7
Tomatoes, cherry	1 cup	11.8
Tomatoes, sun-dried	1 Cup	23.2
Turnips, cooked	1 cup	0.2
Turnip greens, raw	1 cup	138.1
Watercress, raw	1 cup	85.0]
Zucchini, cooked	1 cup	7.6

Fruits		
Apple, with peel	1 medium	3.0
Apple, peeled	1 medium	0.8
Applesauce	1 cup	1.5
Avocado	1/4	10.5
Banana	1 medium	0.6
Blackberries	1 cup	28.5

Blueberries	1 cup	28.0
Cantaloupe, cubed	1 cup	4.0
Cherries, no pits	1 cup	3.0
Cranberries, dried	1/3 cup	1.5
Cranberries, raw	1/3 cup	1.9
Currants	1/2 cup	0
Grapes, red/green, seedless	1 cup	23.4
Kiwi fruit	1 medium	30.6
Lemon	1 medium	0
Lime	1 medium	0
Mango	1 cup	6.9
Melon, cantaloupe, diced	1 cup	3.9
Melon, honeydew, diced	1 cup	4.9
Orange	1 medium	0
Orange peel	1 tsp.	0
Peach	1 medium	2.5
Pear	1 medium	7.5
Pineapple, fresh, diced	1 cup	1.1
Plum	1 each	4.2
Prunes, dried	2 each	10.0
Pumpkin, canned	1 cup	39.2
Raisins	½ cup	2.5
Strawberries, fresh, sliced	1 cup	3.2
Watermelon, fresh, cubed	1 cup	0.2
Meats		
Bacon, pork, cooked	2 strips	0
Beef, cooked, lean	3.5 ounces	1.5
Beef, ground, fried, lean	3.5 ounces	1.4
Beef stock	1 cup	0.2
Chicken, cooked, breast, no skin	3.5 ounces	0.3
Chicken stock	1 cup	0.5
Clams, canned, chopped	1 can	0.3
Clams, fresh	3.5 ounces	0
Crabmeat, cooked	1 cup	0.1
Fish, cod, cooked	3.5 ounces	0.1
Fish, grouper, cooked	3.5 ounces	0
Fish, haddock, cooked	3.5 ounces	0
Fish, halibut, cooked	3.5 ounces	0
Fish, salmon, cooked	3.5 ounces	0
Fish, sole, cooked	3.5 ounces	0.1
Fish, tuna, cooked	3.5 ounces	0
Fish, tuna, canned	3.5 ounces	2.5
Lamb, cooked	3.5 ounces	0

Liver, beef, cooked	3.5 ounces	3.3
Mussels, cooked	3.5 ounces	0
Pork, cooked	3.5 ounces	0
Scallops, cooked	3.5 ounces	0.2
Shrimp, cooked	3.5 ounces	0
Turkey, cooked, no skin	3.5 ounces	0
Turkey pepperoni	3.5 ounces	0
Turkey sausage, cooked	3.5 ounces	1.5

Starches

Bagel	1 whole	0
Biscuit	1	0
Bread, white/wheat/rye	1 slice	0.8
Bulgar, cooked	1 cup	0.9
Cornbread	1 piece – 2.5 x 2.5-inch	0
Cornmeal, blue	100 grams	0
Cornmeal, yellow	1 cup	0.4
Cornstarch	1 cup	0
Couscous, cooked	1 cup	0.2
Crackers, saltine	4 squares	0
Crackers, graham	2 squares	0.8
Croutons, plain	1 cup	0
English muffin	1	0
Flour	1cup	0.4
Grits, cooked	1 cup	0
Melba toast, plain	1 cup, rounds	0.3
Pasta, dry	1 oz	0
Rice, white & brown, cooked	1 cup	0
Rice, wild, cooked	1 cup	0.8
Tortilla, corn, 6-inch	1 each	0
Tortilla, flour, 6-inch	1 each	1.0

Cereals

Barley, dry	1/4 cup	1.0
Cereal, oatmeal	1 cup	1.2
Cereal, cream of wheat	1 cup	0.3
Grits, cooked	1 cup	0

Legumes and Beans		
Almonds	1 oz	0
Bean sprouts, mungo, fresh	1 cup	34.3
Beans, black, dried, cooked	1 cup	0
Beans, garbanzo, canned	1 cup	0
Beans, great northern, dried, cooked	1 cup	0
Beans, great northern, canned	1 cup	0
Beans, kidney, dried, cooked	1 cup	14.9
Beans, kidney, canned	1 cup	5.6
Beans, red kidney, dried, cooked	1 cup	5.8
Beans, red kidney, canned	1 cup	10.5
Beans, lima, dried, cooked	1 cup	3.8
Beans, navy, dried, cooked	1 cup	1.1
Beans, navy, canned	1 cup	7.6
Beans, pinto, dried, cooked	1 cup	6.0
Beans, pinto, canned	1 cup	5.3
Cashews	1/2 cup	23.8
Lentils, dry, cooked	1/4 cup	3.4
Peanuts	2 Tbsp	0
Peanut butter, low fat	1/4 cup	0
Pecans, chopped	1 cup	3.8
Pine nuts	1 oz	15.3
Pistachio nuts	1 cup	0
Soybeans (ddamame)	1 cup	87.4
Tahini	1 Tbsp	0
Tofu	3.5 oz	0
Walnuts, chopped	1 cup	3.2

Dairy		
Buttermilk, non-fat	1 cup	0.2
Cheese, blue	1 oz	0.7
Cheese, cheddar	1 oz	0.8
Cheese, cheddar, reduced fat	1 oz	0.2
Cheese, cottage	1 cup	0.9
Cheese, feta	1 oz	0.5
Cheese, fontina	1 oz	0.7

Cheese, goat	1 oz	0.7
Cheese, monteray	1 oz	0.7
Cheese, mozzarella, part skim	1 oz	0.4
Cheese, parmesan	1 oz	0.5
Cheese, ricotta, reduced fat	1 cup	1.7
Cheese, swiss, low fat	1 oz	1.7
Egg, whole, large	1 each	0.1
Egg, white, large	1 each	0
Egg, yolk large	1 each	0.1
Egg substitute	1 cup	2.0
Milk, 2 percent	1 cup	0.2
Milk, dry, non-fat	1 cup	0.1
Milk, coconut	1 cup	0
Milk, evaporated, non-fat	1 cup	0
Milk, dry, non fat	1 cup	0.1
Milk, soy	1 cup	7.3
Milk, whole	1 cup	0.5
Sour cream, non fat	1 cup	0
Yogurt, plain, low-fat	1 cup	0.5
Beverages		
Beer	12 oz	0
Bourbon	1 oz	0
Carbonated soda	12 oz	0
Coffee, brewed	1 cup	0.2
Coffee, instant, granules	1 tsp	0
Grapefruit juice	1 cup	0
Lemon juice	1 oz	0
Lime juice	1 oz	0.2
Orange juice	1 cup	0.2
Sake	1 oz	0
Tea, brewed	1 cup	0
Tomato juice, canned, no salt	1 cup	5.6
V-8 juice	1 cup	12.8
Vodka	1 oz	0
Wine	1 cup	0
Fats		
Butter	1 tsp.	0.3
Cream cheese	1 Tbsp.	0.4

Mayonnaise, reduced calorie	1 Tbsp.	3.6
Oil, canola	1 tsp.	5.5
Oil, corn	1 tsp.	0.1
Oil, grapeseed	1 tsp.	0
Oil, olive	1 tsp.	2.7
Oil, peanut	1 tsp.	0
Oil, safflower	1 tsp.	0.3
Oil, sesame	1 tsp.	0.6
Oil, soybean	1 tsp.	8.9
Sour cream	1 Tbsp.	0.1

Misc.		
Allspice	1 tsp	0
Baking powder	1 tsp	0
Baking soda	1 tsp	0
Basil, fresh	5 leaves	10.4
Bay leaves, crushed	1 tsp	0
Capers	1 Tbsp	2.1
Cardamom, ground	1 tsp	0
Celery Seed	1 tsp	0
Chili powder	1 tsp	2.7
Chives	1 Tbsp	6.4
Cilantro, fresh	9 sprigs	62.0
Cinnamon, ground	1 tsp	0.7
Cloves, ground	1 tsp	3.0
Cumin, seed	1 tsp	0.1
Curry powder	1 tsp	2.0
Dill, fresh	5 sprigs	0
Garlic powder	1 tsp	0
Gelatin, dry, unflavored	1 envelope	0
Ginger, ground	1 tsp	0
Ginger root	1 tsp	0
Ketchup	1 Tbsp	0.3
Marjoram, ground	1 tsp	3.7
Mint	2 Tbsp	0
Mustard	1 Tbsp	0.4
Mustard, seed	1 tsp	0.2
Nutmeg, ground	1 tsp	0
Olives, ripe, canned	3.5 oz	1.4
Oregano, dried	1 tsp	6.2
Paprika	1 tsp	1.7
Pepper	1 tsp	3.4
Pepper, red, ground	1 tsp	1.4